Integrating Technology into 21st Century Psychiatry: Telemedicine, Social Media, and other Technologies

Editor

JAY H. SHORE

PSYCHIATRIC CLINICS OF NORTH AMERICA

www.psych.theclinics.com

Consulting Editor
HARSH K. TRIVEDI

December 2019 • Volume 42 • Number 4

ELSEVIER

1600 John F. Kennedy Boulevard • Suite 1800 • Philadelphia, Pennsylvania, 19103-2899

http://www.theclinics.com

PSYCHIATRIC CLINICS OF NORTH AMERICA Volume 42, Number 4
December 2019 ISSN 0193-953X, ISBN-13: 978-0-323-70896-8

Editor: Lauren Boyle
Developmental Editor: Kristen Helm

Psychiatric Clinics of North America (ISSN 0193-953X) is published quarterly by Elsevier Inc., 360 Park Avenue South, New York, NY 10010-1710. Months of issue are March, June, September, and December. Business and Editorial Offices: 1600 John F. Kennedy Blvd., Suite 1800, Philadelphia, PA 19103-2899. Periodicals postage paid at New York, NY and additional mailing offices. Subscription prices are $332.00 per year (US individuals), $699.00 per year (US institutions), $100.00 per year (US students/residents), $406.00 per year (Canadian individuals), $462.00 per year (international individuals), $880.00 per year (Canadian & international institutions), and $220.00 per year (Canadian & international students/residents). Foreign air speed delivery is included in all *Clinics*' subscription prices. All prices are subject to change without notice. **POSTMASTER:** Send address changes to *Psychiatric Clinics of North America*, Elsevier Health Sciences Division, Subscription Customer Service, 3251 Riverport Lane, Maryland Heights, MO 63043. **Customer Service: 1-800-654-2452 (US). From outside the United States, call 1-314-447-8871. Fax: 1-314-447-8029. E-mail: journalscustomerservice-usa@elsevier.com (for print support) and journalsonline support-usa@elsevier.com (for online support).**

Reprints. For copies of 100 or more, of articles in this publication, please contact the Commercial Reprints Department, Elsevier Inc., 360 Park Avenue South, New York, New York 10010-1710. Tel.: 212-633-3874, Fax: 212-633-3820, E-mail: reprints@elsevier.com.

Psychiatric Clinics of North America is covered in *MEDLINE/PubMed (Index Medicus)*, *Current Contents/Social and Behavioral Sciences*, *Social Science Citation Index*, *Embase/Excerpta Medica,* and PsycINFO.

Printed in the United States of America.

Contributors

CONSULTING EDITOR

HARSH K. TRIVEDI, MD, MBA
President and Chief Executive Officer, Sheppard Pratt Health System, Baltimore, Maryland

EDITOR

JAY H. SHORE, MD, MPH
Professor, Department of Psychiatry and Family Medicine, School of Medicine, Centers for American Indian and Alaska Native Health, Colorado School of Public Health and Director of Telemedicine Helen and Arthur E. Johnson Depression Center, University of Colorado Anschutz Medical Campus, Aurora, Colorado

AUTHORS

AMBER B. AMSPOKER, PhD
Assistant Professor, VA HSR&D Center for Innovations in Quality, Effectiveness and Safety, Michael E. DeBakey VA Medical Center, (MEDVAMC 152), Baylor College of Medicine, Houston, Texas

DERRECKA BOYKIN, PhD
Instructor, Department of Psychiatry and Behavioral Sciences, Baylor College of Medicine, Postdoctoral Fellow, VA South Central Mental Illness Research, Education and Clinical Center (a Virtual Center), Michael E. DeBakey VA Medical Center, Houston, Texas

ROBERT CAUDILL, MD
Professor, Department of Psychiatry and Behavioral Sciences, University of Louisville, School of Medicine, UofL Physicians Outpatient Center, Louisville, Kentucky

STEVEN CHAN, MD, MBA
Palo Alto Veterans Affairs Health System, Palo Alto, California; Division of Hospital Medicine, Clinical Informatics, University of California, San Francisco, San Francisco, California; Department of Psychiatry, University of California, Davis, Davis, California

EMILY E. CHASCO, PhD
Assistant Research Scientist, Department of Internal Medicine, University of Iowa Roy J. and Lucille A. Carver College of Medicine, Iowa City, Iowa

GISELLE DAY, MPH
Research Associate, VA South Central Mental Illness Research, Education and Clinical Center (a Virtual Center), VA HSR&D Center for Innovations in Quality, Effectiveness and Safety, Michael E. DeBakey VA Medical Center, (MEDVAMC 152), Houston, Texas

STEPHANIE C. DAY, PhD
Assistant Professor, VA South Central Mental Illness Research, Education and Clinical Center (a Virtual Center), Baylor College of Medicine, Houston, Texas

LILIAN N. DINDO, PhD
Michael E. DeBakey VA Medical Center, VHA Health Services Research and Development Center, Department of Medicine, Section of Health Services Research, Baylor College of Medicine, Houston, Texas

ANTHONY H. ECKER, PhD
Investigator, Houston VA HSR&D Center for Innovations in Quality, Effectiveness and Safety, Michael E. DeBakey VA Medical Center (MEDVAMC 152), Instructor, Department of Psychiatry and Behavioral Sciences, Baylor College of Medicine, Investigator, VA South Central Mental Illness Research, Education and Clinical Center (a Virtual Center), Department of Veterans Affairs, Houston, Texas

BRADFORD L. FELKER, MD
VA Puget Sound Health Care System, Seattle Division, Department of Psychiatry and Behavioral Sciences, University of Washington, Seattle, Washington

TERRI L. FLETCHER, PhD
Investigator, Houston VA HSR&D Center for Innovations in Quality, Effectiveness and Safety, Michael E. DeBakey VA Medical Center (MEDVAMC 152), Assistant Professor, Department of Psychiatry and Behavioral Sciences, Baylor College of Medicine, Investigator, VA South Central Mental Illness Research, Education and Clinical Center (a Virtual Center), Department of Veterans Affairs, Houston, Texas

LINDSEY A. FUHRMEISTER, BA
Research Associate, Department of Veterans Affairs, Office of Rural Health Rural Resource Center, Department of Psychiatry, University of Iowa Roy J. and Lucille A. Carver College of Medicine, Iowa City, Iowa

DAVID GRATZER, MD
Centre for Addiction and Mental Health, University of Toronto, Toronto, Ontario

RYAN HAYS, BS
Division of Digital Psychiatry, Department of Psychiatry, Beth Israel Deaconess Medical Center, Harvard Medical School, Boston, Massachusetts

ASHLEY HELM, MA
Research Associate, VA South Central Mental Illness Research, Education and Clinical Center (a Virtual Center), VA HSR&D Center for Innovations in Quality, Effectiveness and Safety, Michael E. DeBakey VA Medical Center, (MEDVAMC 152), Houston, Texas

VICTORIA HENDEL, BA
Division of Digital Psychiatry, Department of Psychiatry, Beth Israel Deaconess Medical Center, Harvard Medical School, Boston, Massachusetts

PHILIP HENSON, MS
Division of Digital Psychiatry, Department of Psychiatry, Beth Israel Deaconess Medical Center, Harvard Medical School, Boston, Massachusetts

JULIANNA HOGAN, PhD
Investigator, Houston VA HSR&D Center for Innovations in Quality, Effectiveness and Safety, Michael E. DeBakey VA Medical Center (MEDVAMC 152), Assistant Professor, Department of Psychiatry and Behavioral Sciences, Baylor College of Medicine,

Investigator, VA South Central Mental Illness Research, Education and Clinical Center (a Virtual Center), Department of Veterans Affairs, Houston, Texas

SHABANA KHAN, MD
Director of Telepsychiatry, Assistant Professor, Department of Child and Adolescent Psychiatry, Hassenfeld Children's Hospital at NYU Langone Health, New York, New York

DAWN M. KLEIN, MSW
Research Manager, Department of Veterans Affairs, Office of Rural Health Rural Resource Center, Department of Psychiatry, University of Iowa Roy J. and Lucille A. Carver College of Medicine, Iowa City, Iowa

LUMING LI, MD
Department of Psychiatry, Yale School of Medicine, Yale University, New Haven, Connecticut

JAN A. LINDSAY, PhD
Investigator, Houston VA HSR&D Center for Innovations in Quality, Effectiveness and Safety, Michael E. DeBakey VA Medical Center (MEDVAMC152), Associate Professor, Department of Psychiatry and Behavioral Sciences, Baylor College of Medicine, Investigator, VA South Central Mental Illness Research, Education and Clinical Center (a Virtual Center), Department of Veterans Affairs, Houston, Texas

JOHN LUO, MD
Chief Medical Information Officer, University of California Riverside School of Medicine, Riverside, California

LINDSEY A. MARTIN, PhD
Assistant Professor, VA HSR&D Center for Innovations in Quality, Effectiveness and Safety, Michael E. DeBakey VA Medical Center, (MEDVAMC 152), Baylor College of Medicine, Houston, Texas

RUSSELL A. McCANN, PhD
Department of Psychiatry and Behavioral Sciences, University of Washington School of Medicine, Seattle, Washington; VA Puget Sound Health Care System, American Lake Division, Lakewood, Washington

MEGHAN M. McGINN, PhD
VA Puget Sound Health Care System, Seattle Division, Department of Psychiatry and Behavioral Sciences, University of Washington School of Medicine, Seattle, Washington

MATTHEW C. MISHKIND, PhD
Assistant Professor, Departments of Family Medicine and Psychiatry, Deputy Director, Johnson Depression Center, University of Colorado School of Medicine, Aurora, Colorado

JOSHUA R. MOORE, MD
Instructor, Department of Psychiatry and Behavioral Sciences, University of Louisville, School of Medicine, UofL Physicians Outpatient Center, Louisville, Kentucky

KEISUKE NAKAGAWA, MD
Postdoctoral Fellow in Physician Health and Well-Being, Department of Psychiatry and Behavioral Sciences, UC Davis Health, Sacramento, California

UJJWAL RAMTEKKAR, MD, MBA, MPE
Associate Medical Director, Partners for Kids (ACO), Assistant Professor, Division of Child and Adolescent Psychiatry, Nationwide Children's Hospital, Ohio State University, Columbus, Ohio

SASHA M. ROJAS, MS
VA Puget Sound Health Care System, Seattle Division, Seattle, Washington; University of Arkansas, Fayetteville, Arkansas

MILENA S. ROUSSEV, PhD
VA Puget Sound Health Care System, Seattle Division, Seattle, Washington

CHRISTOPHER D. SCHNECK, MD
Medical Director, Helen and Arthur E. Johnson Depression Center, Behavioral Health Director, University of Colorado Hospital Infectious Disease/HIV Group Practice, Associate Professor of Psychiatry, Department of Psychiatry and Family Medicine, University of Colorado Anschutz Medical Campus, Aurora, Colorado

ERIKA M. SHEARER, PhD
VA Puget Sound Health Care System, Seattle, Washington; VA Puget Sound Health Care System, American Lake Division, Lakewood, Washington

JAY H. SHORE, MD, MPH
Professor, Department of Psychiatry and Family Medicine, School of Medicine, Centers for American Indian and Alaska Native Health, Colorado School of Public Health and Director of Telemedicine Helen and Arthur E. Johnson Depression Center, University of Colorado Anschutz Medical Campus, Aurora, Colorado

MELINDA A. STANLEY, PhD
Professor Emeritus, Baylor College of Medicine, Houston, Texas

JOHN TOROUS, MD, MBI
Division of Digital Psychiatry, Department of Psychiatry, Beth Israel Deaconess Medical Center, Harvard Medical School, Boston, Massachusetts

CAROLYN L. TURVEY, PhD
Professor, Department of Psychiatry, University of Iowa Roy J. and Lucille A. Carver College of Medicine, Department of Veterans Affairs, Office of Rural Health Rural Resource Center, Iowa City, Iowa

ADITYA VAIDYAM, MS
Division of Digital Psychiatry, Department of Psychiatry, Beth Israel Deaconess Medical Center, Harvard Medical School, Boston, Massachusetts

HANNAH WISNIEWSKI, BS
Division of Digital Psychiatry, Department of Psychiatry, Beth Israel Deaconess Medical Center, Harvard Medical School, Boston, Massachusetts

PETER M. YELLOWLEES, MBBS, MD
Professor of Psychiatry and Vice Chair for Faculty Development, Department of Psychiatry and Behavioral Sciences, Chief Wellness Officer, UC Davis Health, Sacramento, California

Contents

Telemental health is a demonstrated and effective aspect of the overall mental health system and considered a standard of care for many treatments. Adoption has not been as robust as expected and failure to properly develop implementation plans is a significant barrier. This article provides an overview of a step-by-step planning process to more effectively implement and sustain telemental health programs.

Telepsychiatry is used to deliver care to children and adolescents in a variety of settings. Limited literature exists on telepsychiatry education and training, and the vast majority does not address considerations unique to practicing telepsychiatry with youth. Without relevant education, clinical experience, and exposure to technology, child and adolescent psychiatrists may be resistant to integrating telepsychiatry into their practice. Additional research is needed to assess the current state of telepsychiatry education and training in child and adolescent psychiatry fellowship programs.

This article describes the Personalized Implementation for Video Telehealth strategy to increase adoption of video telehealth to home (VTH) across a large, urban Veterans Health Administration medical center and applications for broader use in non-VHA settings. The authors fully integrated VTH into existing mental health clinics, resulting in (1) a significant increase in the number of patients receiving VTH, (2) a significant increase in the number of VTH visits relative to median national improvement, (3) a greater number of unique specialty mental health clinics offering VTH in Houston, and (4) a greater number of community clinics active in delivering VTH.

Video-to-home (VTH) is a patient-centered approach to delivering mental health care that has increased the reach of care to patients who face considerable logistical and sociocultural barriers. Despite high rates of patient satisfaction and acceptance of VTH, scholarly resources for expanding providers' comfort and competence using VTH are limited to emergency preparedness or remotely managing higher risk patients. This article highlights other potential benefits, adaptations, and considerations for providers interested in expanding their use of VTH to engage patients who are difficult to reach or who have complex presentations.

There is increasing evidence that the delivery of mental health services via clinical video telehealth (CVT) is an effective means of providing services to individuals with access barriers, such as rurality. However, many providers have concerns about working with individuals at risk for suicide via this modality, and many clinical trials have excluded individuals with suicide risk factors. The present article reviews the literature, professional guidelines, and laws that pertain to the provision of mental health services via CVT with high-risk patients and provides suggestions for adapting existing best-practice recommendations for assessing and managing suicide risk to CVT delivery.

Self-help and automated technologies can be useful for behavioral and mental health education and interventions. These technologies include interactive media, online courses, artificial intelligence–powered chatbots, voice assistants, and video games. Self-help media can include books, videos, audible media like podcasts, blog and print articles, and self-contained Internet sites. Social media, online courses, and mass-market mobile apps also can include such media. These technologies serve to decrease geospatial, temporal, and financial barriers. This article describes different self-help and automated technologies, how to implement such technologies in existing clinical services, and how to implement according to patient needs.

Traditionally, the assessment of cognition and the administration of cognitive therapies has been performed in the clinic, but with modern technology, this clinic-centric view is changing. This article explores the landscape of digital devices used to measure cognition in settings outside the clinic. These devices range in mobility from user-friendly mobile devices to setting-specific devices able to provide powerful, robust cognitive therapy and living assistance in the comfort of a patient's home. Although these methods remain in early stages of developmental, initial studies suggest they may prove useful in treating patients with serious mental illnesses in a widespread clinical setting.

The goal of automating complex human activities dates to antiquity. The mental health field has also made use of advances in technology to assist patients in need. Artificial Intelligence (AI) is the study of agents that receive percepts from the environment and perform actions. AI is increasingly being incorporated into the development of chatbots that can be deployed in both clinical and nonclinical settings. Chatbots are a computer program that simulates human conversation through voice commands or text chats or both. The collaboration between AI therapists and more traditional providers of such care will only grow.

Electronic health records combined with tethered patient portals now support a range of functions including electronic data capture of patient-reported outcomes, trend reporting on clinical targets, secure messaging, and patient-mediated health information exchange. The applications of these features require special consideration in psychiatric and behavioral health settings. Nonetheless, their potential to engage patients suffering from disorders in which passivity and withdrawal are endemic to their mental health condition, is great. This article presents the growing research base on these topics, including discussion of key issues and recommendations for optimal implementation of patient portals in behavioral health settings.

The Internet is a vast expanse of information; however, search engines have made finding the proverbial needle in a haystack a simple matter. Although insurance provider databases and referrals may dominate how patients find their doctor today, one's online reputation and reviews on physician ratings sites will increasingly play a role in how prospective patients find their next provider. Social media plays a dominant role as the medium where people place and find information, blurring the boundary of professional and personal use. Privacy online has become an endangered species, requiring active strategies to keep it from going extinct.

Culture plays a critical role in shaping the structure, content, and process of psychiatric treatment and influences the use of technology. Mental health providers and health care systems should account for the impact of the interface of technology and culture on clinical processes. Psychiatrists need to assess and monitor the impact of this interface on therapeutic processes. Health care systems should attend to these issues as they develop, adapt, and deploy technologies. As a field, psychiatry needs to develop frameworks for formally evaluating the use of existing and innovating technologies for use in mental health treatment.

Technology is increasingly being incorporated into the everyday workflows of physicians. There are concerns that electronic medical records and other digital technologies will contribute to the growing epidemic of physician burnout. However, some technologies, such as telemedicine, have demonstrated positive effects on physician health by saving time, enhancing work-life balance, improving quality, and restoring more control and flexibility to their practices. Organizations often lack data to evaluate the impact of technologies on physician health. The University of California Technology Wellness Index is a framework that provides a fast, systematic, physician-centered method to assess the impact of technology on physician well-being.

PSYCHIATRIC CLINICS OF NORTH AMERICA

SERIES OF RELATED INTEREST

Child and Adolescent Psychiatric Clinics of North America
https://www.childpsych.theclinics.com/

Neurologic Clinics
https://www.neurologic.theclinics.com/

THE CLINICS ARE AVAILABLE ONLINE!
Access your subscription at:
www.theclinics.com

PSYCHIATRIC CLINICS OF NORTH AMERICA

FORTHCOMING ISSUES

March 2020
Mixed Affective States Beyond Current
Boundaries
Alan C. Swann and Gabriele Sani, Editors

June 2020
Neuropsychiatry
Vassilis E. Koliatsos, Editor

September 2020
Achieving Mental Health Equity
Altha Stewart and Ruth Shim, Editors

RECENT ISSUES

September 2019
Professional Development for Psychiatrists
Howard Y. Liu and Donald M. Hilty, Editors

June 2019
Eating Disorders: Part II
Harry A. Brandt and Steven F. Crawford,
Editors

March 2019
Eating Disorders: Part I
Harry A. Brandt and Steven F. Crawford,
Editors

SERIES OF RELATED INTEREST

Child and Adolescent Psychiatric Clinics of North America
http://www.childpsych.theclinics.com

Neurologic Clinics
http://www.neurologic.theclinics.com

THE CLINICS ARE AVAILABLE ONLINE!
Access your subscription at:
www.theclinics.com

Preface

Welcome to the Era of Continuous Practice Transformation

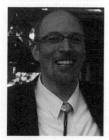

Jay H. Shore, MD, MPH
Editor

We are at an unprecedented historical moment in the history of technological transformation of society. The changes birthed at the end of the twentieth century have accelerated to an exponential pace permeating all aspects of personal and professional life, including medicine and psychiatry. Technology in all its forms has become an integral part of psychiatric practice, precipitating an era of continuous practice adaptation and transformation. For both the individual provider and behavioral health organizations, keeping abreast of these changes can be daunting. The intent of this issue of *Psychiatric Clinics of North America* is to provide a pragmatic review of some of the major technologies being used in psychiatric practice as well as those on the near horizon that are likely to contribute to the next wave of practice transformation. An additional aim is to help providers integrate and adapt these technologies into their practices and gain an understanding of the strengths and limitations of technologies used in clinical settings.

The issue begins with a series of articles focused on Telepsychiatry in the form of videoconferencing, which is one of the more mature technologies that was piloted initially in the late 1950s. Today, Telepsychiatry has progressed to widespread utilization and dissemination through adaptation to smaller and more nimble platforms. Currently it enables the provision of care directly to the patient's location whether clinic, office, or home. We then turn to a broader array of technologies, several in nascent phases of clinical deployment, and explore the current and future potential impacts and consequences of their use.

Dr Mishkind leads off the issue with a "how-to" approach for developing and implementing videoconferencing services, followed by an overview by Drs Kahn and Ramtekkar on Telepsychiatry with child and adolescent populations with accompanying key resources. The issue then focuses on the growth of mobile videoconferencing with an example from Dr Lindsay and her team in organizational

Psychiatr Clin N Am 42 (2019) xiii–xiv
https://doi.org/10.1016/j.psc.2019.08.012
0193-953X/19/© 2019 Published by Elsevier Inc.

psych.theclinics.com

implemenation, proffering distilled recommendations for others undertaking the development of these services. Dr Hogan and colleagues share lessons learned in mobile videoconferencing, using challenging cases to explore important clinical issues that arise in the treatment of patients in nonclinical settings. The foci on mobile videoconferencing concludes with perspectives on managing high-risk suicidal patients.

The technological scope is broadened with a review of self-help and automated tools in mental health care. The theme is expanded upon with an article surveying the developing technology for cognitive assessment of psychiatric disorders, followed by Drs Moore and Caudill's review of interactive computer treatments that are evolving into the promise of fully autonomous BOT-driven psychiatric interventions. The attention on automation finishes with a consideration of how data being captured in electronic health records and patient portals can be leveraged to support behavioral health.

The final section does not concentrate on specfic technologies or technology-driven processes, but rather on implications of technology and technology practice transformation on physicians. Dr Luo grants guidance for psychiatrists on best practices for managing one's online reputation, which is an area of concern developing over the past decade, as the Internet has become a key enabler of sociatal interactions. The impact of intended and unintended consequences as technology and culture collide in psychiatric treatment is considerable, and a proffered framework helps providers navigate these issues. We conclude with a tool proposed by Drs Nakagawa and Yellowlees, The University of California Technology Wellness Index (UCTWI), to assess the use of technologies to support the emerging field of physician health and wellness. Physician care is an appropriate topic on which to conclude, as all physicians and providers seek to achieve personal and professional balance in the midst of this unprecendented technological transformation.

Jay H. Shore, MD, MPH
Department of Psychiatry and
Family Medicine
School of Medicine
Centers for American Indian and Alaska Native Health
Colorado School of Public Health
Telemedicine Helen and
Arthur E. Johnson Depression Center
University of Colorado
Anschutz Medical Campus
Mail Stop F800
13055 East 17th Avenue
Aurora, CO 80045, USA

E-mail address:
jay.shore@cuanschutz.edu

Establishing Telemental Heath Services from Conceptualization to Powering up

Matthew C. Mishkind, PhD

KEYWORDS

- Telemental health planning • Needs assessment • Sustain services

KEY POINTS

- Telemental health is an effective aspect of the overall health care system.
- Adoption and sustainment of services is often lower than expected.
- Failure to properly plan for program implementation and ongoing sustainment leads to program failures.

INTRODUCTION

The new information age in which we live is an exciting time to be a part of mental health care, as advances in telecommunications technologies have made it increasingly possible to provide and receive a range of safe and effective mental health services that reach beyond traditional clinical settings. Telemental health (TMH), which is the use of technology to provide mental health care services at a geographic or temporal distance, has increased in acceptance and utilization.[1] This excitement and increased acceptance can lead to an impression that technology is the solution to many concerns about health care systems, including access to service, increased quality of care, reduced stigma to seeking care, and more efficient use of health resources.[2–4] This is due in part to raised awareness about the benefits of TMH and because many of the technologies and peripherals used to deliver services today are ubiquitous to consumers based largely on commercial use and applications. For example, synchronous audio-visual connections used to require stand-alone video-conference equipment and can now be done with minimal network drops through built-in smartphone applications.

Disclosure Statement: N/A.
Departments of Family Medicine and Psychiatry, Johnson Depression Center, University of Colorado School of Medicine, 13199 East Montview Boulevard, Suite 330, Aurora, CO 80045, USA
E-mail address: Matthew.mishkind@ucdenver.edu

Psychiatr Clin N Am 42 (2019) 545–554
https://doi.org/10.1016/j.psc.2019.08.002
0193-953X/19/© 2019 Elsevier Inc. All rights reserved.

TMH has proved to be an effective aspect of the overall mental health system and a standard of care for many mental health concerns. However, the promise of TMH has not been met with broad-based implementation success.[5] This is due in part to program planning failures that too often begin with finding a use for technology rather than using technology to meet a need.[6,7] Other planning issues can focus on not understanding patient populations and the willingness or capacity of staff to deliver new services. Finally, technology evolves much faster than policy and programs can fail when they do not fit within existing regulatory environments.

The purpose of this article is to provide an overview of steps necessary to conceive of, develop, implement, and ultimately sustain a program. Although these steps are provided as a step-by-step guide for organizational simplicity, many, if not all, can be done concurrently. This paper is not an official guideline and therefore none of the language should be taken as a regulatory requirement. Rather, it is meant as a guide to assist program developers and with the broader adoption of TMH services. The first step to developing a program should begin with a needs assessment well before any services are initiated.

CONDUCT A NEEDS ASSESSMENT—UNDERSTAND THE PROBLEM TO BE SOLVED

Programs tend to fail to launch effectively or experience later critical issues when planners do not properly understand the problem that TMH is attempting to solve.[8] Evaluating the needs for a TMH solution should form the foundation of any program and is recommended as a critical step in program success.[9] Although the initial decisions derived from a needs assessment can be modified, it is important to begin with a solid and realistic foundation about why TMH is needed, who it will serve, and how it will serve them.

A recent joint guideline between the American Telemedicine Association and American Psychiatric Association (ATA-APA) notes that a needs assessment should be conducted before initiating services.[10] An important first question to answer is related to the overall intent of a new TMH service. For example, is the program intended to provide convenience for current patients, increase access for at-risk patient populations, or serve as an opportunity to broaden market scope and share? For some it may be that TMH is a way to stay competitive in a specific market. There is no fundamentally right or wrong answer assuming it fits the situation and problem to be solved. An overview of 5 initial steps to help identify your base program needs follows.

STEP 1: DEVELOP A PROGRAM STATEMENT

The ultimate goal of a needs assessment is to define what the ATA-APA guidelines refer to as a "Program Overview Statement." This is a simple, straightforward purpose statement about the problem to be solved based on results of the needs assessment. This statement should provide an initial, operationalized overview of the program that can be used to socialize development plans to stakeholders, drive future program decisions, and evaluate program effectiveness. The statement is best finalized after all data have been collected and analyzed. However, a working statement can be drafted once the following components, at a minimum, are understood.

Proposed Patient Population

Planners will likely already have an idea of potential at-need patients or new legislation and policies that afford new opportunities for TMH care. Maintaining awareness of ongoing service needs and trends is the best place to start. However, to truly understand your proposed patient population requires not just an understanding of needs but also an understanding of whether your intended population will elect to access the services you want to provide. Successful TMH programs start with taking a deep look at the needs of the local community focusing on the barriers to health care access and the reasons that patients are at high risk. Some sample questions to ask at this stage of the process include the following:

- What health care concerns do you feel are not being adequately addressed in the existing clinic, and will TMH help?
- What do you see as the greatest health care access challenges?
- What steps, successful or not, have already been taken to address these concerns, and are there options other than TMH?
- Will patients use any technology-based services that may be offered?
- Any exclusion criteria? If so, what are they? How will they be applied? (eg, does the provider make the call, does the originating site play any role in screening)

Services to be Delivered

Once you understand your patient needs, demographics, and potential for accessing a new program you can evaluate what services to offer. New programs are often most successful when they initially focus on the simplest way to meet patients needs. Remember that programs can build in complexity through iterations of success. It is much more difficult to scale back services because the initial program overshot what could realistically be accomplished. A key recommendation in this step is to start with the most pressing need, show success, and then build the capacity to expand. Sample questions to ask at this stage include the following:

- What services will bridge your most pressing gaps in care?
- How will these services be integrated into existing clinical operations including the option of expanded clinical hours?
- Where do you want to physically provide the services—where will the patients and providers be located?
- What investments (time, personnel, technology, space, supporting services) are you prepared to make in order to expand access to care through telehealth?
- How are you planning to maintain the services?

Draft Program Statement

A sample draft program statement may read as, for example, "The XYZ TMH service will deliver synchronous mental health care to established patients for enhanced continuity of care and ongoing access. It will be offered to new patients with access to care challenges such as mobility concerns or living in underserved areas." Modifications are expected as additional needs assessment data are analyzed and understood. The next step in the process is to understand your existing personnel and technology resources, and any gaps you will likely need to fill.

STEP 2: EVALUATE EXISTING PERSONNEL RESOURCES

Research indicates that patients tend to be initially more accepting of receiving TMH services than providers are of delivering them.[11] For some providers there is additional concern about how best to engage patients and more effectively use technologies to enhance care and maintain patient-provider relationships.[12,13] The next step in the needs assessment process is to determine if you have providers on staff who are able and willing to deliver the planned TMH care services. This should include an understanding of clinic process flows and whether a new program will integrate with or serve as a replacement for existing services and potentially requiring additional staff. Some sample questions to ask include the following:

- Does your staff (providers, administrative, technical etc.) have experience providing TMH services, and are they willing to provide them?
- Do you have the necessary staff to support your clinicians?
- Do you anticipate changes to workflows or additional duties for staff?
- Who will orient the patient to the nature of telehealth and who will go over consent forms (if necessary) with him/her? Who will ensure that the equipment is on and operating properly and that the connection with the provider is made?

STEP 3: MATCH YOUR TECHNOLOGY TO YOUR NEEDS

The services to be provided and the needs of your program should drive the technology. The lure of new, interesting technology may create pressure to plan the technology before appropriately understanding the use cases for it. This can increase the probability that the program will fail due to poor utilization or costs overruns. A technology plan should begin with an evaluation of needs identified in the previous steps with additional focus on the functions needed by the patient and provider. The goal is to develop specifications for the equipment and technology needed to deliver your planned services to your planned patient population as effectively and efficiently as possible. This is also a good place to begin the process of understanding organizational needs and currently available resources, as you may already have access to the necessary technology. Evaluating outside vendor products may be required if the technology is not currently available. Some sample questions to ask during this step of the assessment include the following:

- Are you required by your organization or payors to meet technology specifications?
- Is your preferred technology already available to you and does it meet regulatory specifications such as HIPAA?
- Do you have staff available to maintain and troubleshoot any technology issues during or outside of clinical sessions?
- Will any records be transmitted to the provider before or during the visit?
- Does your medical records system support virtual services?
- How will educational materials that the clinician wishes to provide to the patient be managed? How will "homework" or self-monitoring forms be transmitted to the provider?

STEP 4: DETERMINE YOUR OPERATIONAL SPACE

TMH affords opportunities to deliver services in varied operational spaces including clinically supervised (eg, outpatient mental health clinic) and clinically unsupervised (eg, patient home) settings. In fact, much of the innovation in TMH comes from understanding how to use different spaces given regulatory constraints. Where the patient is located (the originating site) rather than where the provider is located (the distant site) is where care is typically said to be delivered. This affects your operational space because state laws and state licensing authorities have different regulations for clinically supervised and unsupervised settings. Plans for providing services in one jurisdiction will not immediately equate to a similar plan in another location.

An effective way to understand your operational space is to evaluate the step-by-step needs of your program to determine where care can be delivered appropriately. Working through what is likely to be a typical clinical visit is a recommended pathway for this step in the process. This should begin before the encounter and continue through to referrals and other next steps. Following are some sample questions to ask during this step in the process:

- How will patients be referred and know about the service?
- How will appointments be made and how will patients access technologies?
- Will the originating site be incorporated into a clinically supervised setting?
- What will be the process if patients refuse TMH and prefer a face-to-face visit?
- How will privacy and confidentiality concerns be addressed?
- How will the patient be brought physically or virtually into the session and introduced to the provider?
- How will orders resulting from the encounter (laboratories, meds, referrals) be managed?
- What will happen at the end of an encounter?

STEP 5: UNDERSTAND YOUR REGULATORY ENVIRONMENT

State and federal laws and licensing board regulations continue to evolve with many of the changes occurring at the local level. It is critically important to understand the legal and regulatory requirements for your originating and distant site operational spaces. Licensure, credentialing and privileging, and malpractice insurance are often seen as the primary regulatory barriers to implementing TMH services.[12] Although important, there are other less referenced regulations that are equally important to address for a successful program. For example, you will need to comply with the Ryan Haight Act Online Pharmacy Consumer Protection Act (federal law that amended the Controlled Substances Act) if you plan to prescribe controlled substances.[14] Or, if you are an HIPAA-covered entity you will likely need a business associate agreement with your technology vendor to ensure security of protected health information. The following section gives an overview of additional questions to answer about regulatory considerations before initiating services:

- Licensure
  - Are providers licensed where patients are located?
- Malpractice insurance
  - Have you checked to make sure all providers will be covered to provide the services?
- Credentialing and privileging
  - Where are your providers credentialed/where do they have privileges? Do you know the process for telehealth?
- Workload accounting and coding
  - How will you code and document telehealth visits—will you provide different workload credit?
- Emergency procedures
  - Clinically supervised settings: are existing procedures adequate for TMH services?
  - Clinically unsupervised settings: are new procedures such as how to use a Patient Support Person required?
- Informed consent
  - Is an additional consent for TMH required, and if so, does it need to be written?

DEVELOP A PLAN—DRAFT POLICIES, PROCEDURES, AND PROTOCOLS

The results of the needs assessment should provide the information and details necessary to develop an operational plan of local policies, procedures, and protocols. In many situations, the needs assessment serves as the initial draft for your plan and the work at this stage of the process is focused on filling in gaps and developing standard processes and documents that supports the patient, the referring provider, the remote clinic staff, and the local staff. The overriding goal of these documents is to make certain that the scope of TMH practice is equivalent to the care that would otherwise be provided in person.

Many professional associations including the ATA and the APA have written guidelines that should be referenced to assist with document development.[10,15–18] Incorporating additional requirements into already existing documents is recommended to assist implementation; be mindful to not unnecessarily replicate existing procedures. For example, existing emergency procedures in clinically supervised settings may require minimal modifications for TMH services. Translating these documents into approved clinical protocols can be done once a commitment is made to implement a program, and procedures have been tested in practice.

DEVELOP A BUSINESS PLAN—SUSTAIN AND MARKET SERVICES

Reimbursement is often cited as a significant barrier to TMH program implementation and despite most of the states having passed some form of telehealth parity law, it can be difficult to maintain a program based entirely on clinical reimbursements.[17] Medicaid will also reimburse for some services.[19] It is natural to want to start initiating services as quickly as possible, especially after the overall service program has been defined. It is also reasonable to expect that providers and systems do not have an appetite for taking on new services that either do not pay as well or that do pay as well but create other issues such as increased demand without adequate supply. Developing a business plan that understands costs, revenues, and return-on-investment is a critical step that is often omitted but is necessary for sustainability of the program. A recommendation is to develop a sustainment model that uses multiple payment structures.

Identify Funding Models

Your organization or private practice will need to maintain financial viability to continue providing services to your patients. Telehealth should not be a detriment to the financial status of the organization. It should be planned so that its return on investment to the organization will be realized. Practitioners maintaining a private practice may be able to sustain a program through a combination of insurance (including Medicaid and Medicare as appropriate) and private pay. For many this may not be feasible because of low rates of reimbursement, lower than expected demand, and potential for burn-out due to utilization demands. Developing hybrid-partnership models that include grants, contracts, and direct reimbursements may help offset gaps from a single source of revenue. Some models beyond traditional fee-for-service or insurance reimbursements are included here:

- *Grants*: grants are often useful to help initiate programs and obtain up-front funding for technology and personnel. Grants rarely provide sustainment funding.
- *Contracts*: contracting with a partner organization in need of services can be an effective way to sustain operations. This can be accomplished as a direct contract hire or a full-time equivalent buyout to provide specialty services.

- *Partnering with the payer*: it has become more common for providers to directly partner with payers to fulfill a need or even local mandates for access to care.

Develop a Marketing Plan

Although patients express a desire for TMH services, adoption has been slower than expected in part because patients are not aware that services are available. The first marketing step includes communication to leaders of the community, patients, health care providers, and other health care organizations. Depending on the funding model, marketing may include participating in announcements with partner organizations and developing additional alliances to broaden outreach activities. Developing relationships with major local employers and highlighting how the TMH service can assist their employees is a method for reaching captive audiences. Another effective strategy is to develop a referral partnership with other health care disciplines such as local primary care clinics that may be struggling with addressing mental health needs of patients. Finally, develop community training programs that highlight an area of expertise (eg, youth anxiety) and promote the TMH services you offer.

EVALUATE TRAINING NEEDS AND TRAIN STAFF—PREPARE PERSONNEL

Research suggests that providers may be more reluctant to embrace TMH for several reasons including concerns about developing rapport with patients, patient compliance, and less successful treatment outcomes.[11] Many of these concerns may be due to limited training opportunities for providers to better engage with and understand the functional delivery of TMH services. One study found that about half of the providers using TMH felt properly trained to deliver services.[20] As a result, provider training and education tends to be a focal point when implementing a new service. Fortunately, there is evidence to suggest that when given information about the utility of TMH, and provided opportunities to engage service delivery, provider reluctance can be reduced. However, limiting training to providers may hinder the development of a TMH service program. A recommendation is to evaluate the training needs of all program-related staff to understand the various administrative, technical, programmatic, and organizational aspects of the service.

One study implemented and evaluated a training protocol used for a deploying Army unit tasked to expand TMH services in Afghanistan.[21] The training evaluation suggested 5 best practices for training sessions with the goal of providing comprehensive training across all roles and responsibilities. An overview of the best practices follows:

- *First*, identify which topics are best trained in a live setting versus those better suited for didactic learning that may be more efficiently conducted through online and other distant learning media. Some topics more suitable for didactic learning include background, history, and evidence base of TMH.
- *Second*, focus on live, interactive sessions for the practice of trouble-shooting technology issues, practicing rapport-building techniques, and implementing standard operating procedures. It is not the intent of these sessions to turn novices into experts after one session, but rather to give trainees the tools they need to know to begin implementing the program.
- *Third*, use lessons learned from other known programs or research to develop real-to-life training scenarios.
- *Fourth*, incorporate training into daily activities rather than limiting to a training session. For example, rather than conducting a distant work meeting via teleconference, work to set up synchronous audio–video communications to allow

participants to gain additional understanding of the subtleties associated with this form of communication.

- *Fifth,* tailor training based on roles while ensuring that all stakeholders have the same base competencies and knowledge sets. Although it is not necessary or even feasible for all program staff to have the same advanced knowledge across disciplines, it is important to have the same level of base training to self-sufficiently perform necessary TMH roles and duties. Developing this base knowledge of telehealth for all stakeholders should ensure a more common understanding for the uses and benefits of telehealth and related services, which may facilitate further expansion.

The overarching theme is that interactive training in the form of live, simulated clinical and technical scenarios is an invaluable training method. It is likely that training resources are constrained and using data captured in the initial needs assessment (eg, staff experience with TMH) will help tailor a training program for staff. Finally, consider the familiarity that patients have, or not, with TMH and technology in general. Developing a brief pamphlet, or introductory videos, explaining the benefits and procedures of TMH may be necessary to increase patient engagement. An additional recommendation is to conduct short test sessions with patients before an initial TMH session.

DEVELOP AN EVALUATION PLAN—MEASURE WHAT YOU CAN CONTROL

The success of a TMH program can extend far beyond the initially proposed goals. For example, improving access to mental health services has been shown to lead to reductions in hospital visits and other clinical outcomes.[22] It can be rewarding to think about these broader goals and even changes to the overall health care system. However, this level of goal setting can lead to an evaluation plan that is impossible to affect and execute. In fact, developing too many goals is more likely to result in fewer goals being met.

The goal of a TMH program is behavior change in the form of increased access and adoption and improved quality and efficiency of services. Other goals such as policy changes and increased revenue are necessary but insufficient for true change to occur. Several models exist that focus on effective program execution. One model that has proved effective across industries at changing behaviors across different programs is known as the Four Disciplines of Execution.[23] An overview of this model is presented later beginning with a focus on a limited number of Wildly Important Goals:

- *Wildly important goals*: develop no more than 2 to 3 critical goals for your program. These should be executable and directed toward meeting the final outcomes of the program (battles that win the war).
- *Focus on lead indicators*: there is a tendency to focus on lag indicator outcomes such as improved clinical care. Although lag indicators may be the goal of a program, they are not as readily influenced and once they can be measured too much time has passed for quick action. Focus instead on lead indicators that can be influenced and predict outcomes.
- *Keep a scorecard*: scorecards are effective at keeping everyone on the same page. The best scorecards are simple, visible to all, and show immediate results. Remember the saying, "what gets measured gets managed."
- *Create accountability*: develop a system for all stakeholders to identify time-limited action steps and receive immediate feedback.

TEST, EVALUATE, AND MODIFY

Running a TMH program is ultimately a task of sustainment. Regulations change, populations shift, new technologies are developed, and the costs associated with various aspects of a program go up and down. By vigilantly monitoring the different aspects of a program you can see trends before they happen and modify programs before it is necessary. Treat new initiatives as pilots you know going into will require modifications. Learn from evaluations, capture quantitative and qualitative data, and adjust as necessary. Finally, periodically reconsider the steps outlined in this paper to identify important changes.

SUMMARY

The landscape of TMH will continue to evolve with changes in technology, regulations, reimbursement standards, and overall acceptance. The field has already seen shifts from initial pilots to sustainable programs that require broad-scoped planning for success. In addition, the field has seen rapid shifts in what forms the basis of a TMH program from technology driving plans to plans incorporating technology to meet specific needs. As TMH continues to be shown as a standard of care and viable alternative to traditional services, the value of a well-planned and executed planning process focused on broader adoption has become increasingly important.

The importance of planning can be seen in the number of other reference documents and sites that are available. The American Telemedicine Association has several guidelines for TMH practice and as noted earlier the joint ATA-APA guidelines include some best practices for establishing a service. Other available resources include the APA's Telepsychiatry Toolkit (https://www.psychiatry.org/psychiatrists/practice/telepsychiatry/toolkit), the National Consortium of Telehealth Resource Centers (https://www.telehealthresourcecenter.org/), and the ATA (https://www.americantelemed.org/) with specific focus on the ATA Telemental Health Special Interest Group.

This article provides a consolidated reference manual to help understand the general requirements to start a TMH service. It is based on research, practical applications, and real-world experiences developing and creating TMH programs. Although it provides a robust overview, it should be used with other resources including those listed earlier to make certain details are covered in depth. Through planning and sustainment activities, TMH will continue to grow in number of services available and overall adoption rates.

REFERENCES

1. Adams SM, Rice MJ, Jones SL, et al. TeleMental health: standards, reimbursement, and interstate practice. J Am Psychiatr Nurses Assoc 2018;24(4):295–305.
2. Bashshur RL, Shannon GW, Bashshur N, et al. The empirical evidence for telemedicine interventions in mental disorders. Telemed J E Health 2015;22(2):87–113.
3. Hilty DM, Ferrer DC, Parish MB, et al. The effectiveness of telemental health: a 2013 review. Telemed J E Health 2013;19(6):444–54.
4. Hubley S, Lynch SB, Schneck C, et al. Review of key telepsychiatry outcomes. World J Psychiatry 2016;6(2):269–82.
5. Ellimoottil C, An L, Moyer M, et al. Challenges and opportunities faced by large health systems implementing telehealth. Health Aff 2018;37(12):1955–9.

6. Ross J, Stevenson F, Lau R, et al. Factors that influence the implementation of e-Health: a systematic review of systematic reviews (an update). Implement Sci 2016;11(1):146–57.

7. Ross J, Stevenson F, Dack C, et al. Developing an implementation strategy for a digital health intervention: an example in routine healthcare. BMC Health Serv Res 2018;18:794–806.

8. AlDossary S, Martin-Khan MG, Bradford NK, et al. The development of a telemedicine planning framework based on needs assessment. J Med Syst 2017;41: 74–82.

9. DeGaetano N, Shore J. Conducting a telehealth needs assessment. In: Tuerk PW, Shore P, editors. Clinical videoconferencing in telehealth. Switzerland: Springer International Publishing Behavioral Telehealth; 2015. p. 23–54.

10. Shore JH, Yellowlees P, Caudill R, et al. Best practices in videoconferencing-based telemental health. Telemed J E Health 2018;24(11):827–32.

11. Brooks E, Turvey C, Augusterfer EF. Provider barriers to telemental health: obstacles overcome, obstacles remaining. Telemed J E Health 2013;19(6):433–7.

12. Kramer GM, Kinn JT, Mishkind MC. Legal, regulatory, and risk management issues in the use of technology to deliver mental health care. Cogn Behav Pract 2015;22:258–68.

13. Macdonald GG, Townsend AF, Adam P, et al. eHealth technologies, multimorbidity, and the office visit: qualitative interview study on the perspectives of physicians and nurses. J Med Internet Res 2018;20(1):1–12.

14. Mackey TK, Kalyanam J, Katsuki T, et al. Twitter-based detection of illegal online sale of prescription opioid. Am J Public Health 2017;107(12):1910–5.

15. Myers K, Nelson EL, Rabinowitz T, et al. American Telemedicine Association practice guidelines for telemental health with children and adolescents. Telemed J E Health 2017;23(10):779–804.

16. Shore JH, Mishkind MC, Bernard J, et al. A lexicon of assessment and outcome measures for telemental health. Telemed J E Health 2014;23(3):282–92.

17. Turvey C, Coleman M, Dennison O, et al. ATA Practice Guidelines for Video-Based Online Mental Health Services. Telemed J E Health 2013;19(9):722–30.

18. Health policy brief: telehealth parity laws. Health Aff 2016. Available at: http://www.healthaffairs.org/healthpolicybriefs/brief.php?brief_id=162.

19. Fortney JC, Veith RC, Bauer AM, et al. Developing telemental health partnerships between State Medical Schools and Federally Qualified Health Centers: navigating the regulatory landscape and policy recommendations. J Rural Health 2019;35(3):287–97.

20. Jameson JP, Farmer MS, Head KJ, et al. VA Community Mental Health Service providers' utilization of and attitudes toward telemental healthcare: the gatekeeper's perspective. J Rural Health 2011;27:425–32.

21. Mishkind MC, Boyd A, Kramer GM, et al. Evaluating the benefits of a live, simulation-based telebehavioral health training for a deploying army reserve unit. Mil Med 2013;187(12):1322–7.

22. Godleski L, Darkins A, Peters J. Outcomes of 98,609 U.S. Department of Veterans Affairs Patients Enrolled in Telemental Health Services, 2006-2010. Psychiatr Serv 2012;63(4):383–5.

23. McChesney C, Covey S, Huling J. The 4 disciplines of execution: achieving your wildly important goals. New York: Free Press; 2012.

Child and Adolescent Telepsychiatry Education and Training

Shabana Khan, MD[a],*, Ujjwal Ramtekkar, MD, MBA, MPE[b]

KEYWORDS

- Telemedicine • Telepsychiatry • Telemental health • E-health • Telehealth
- Training and education • Child psychiatry

KEY POINTS

- Telepsychiatry education and training are important to ensure successful implementation and sustainability of pediatric telepsychiatry services.
- Limited literature exists on telepsychiatry education and training and the vast majority does not address considerations unique to practicing telepsychiatry with children and adolescents.
- Future directions include developing an evidence-based pediatric telepsychiatry curriculum for trainees and practicing child and adolescent psychiatrists.

INTRODUCTION

Recent data estimate that approximately 11% of children and adolescents in the United States have a serious emotional disturbance with significant functional impairment,[1] and approximately half of adults with psychiatric illness receive their diagnosis before age 15.[2] Despite the availability of effective treatments, a significant percentage of youth with mental health disorders do not receive needed treatment and for those who do, there often is a significant delay from symptom onset to diagnosis and treatment initiation.

One reason for the lack of or delays in treatment is the significant shortage and maldistribution of child and adolescent psychiatrists. These access issues have a disproportionate impact on children and adolescents living outside major metropolitan areas

Disclosure Statement: The authors have nothing to disclose.
[a] Department of Child and Adolescent Psychiatry, Hassenfeld Children's Hospital at NYU Langone Health, One Park Avenue, 7th Floor, New York, NY 10016, USA; [b] Partner for Kids (ACO), Division of Child and Adolescent Psychiatry, Nationwide Children's Hospital/Ohio State University, 700 Children's Drive, T4 Suite A.007, Columbus, OH 43025, USA
* Corresponding author.
E-mail address: Shabana.Khan@nyulangone.org
twitter: @ShabanaKhanMD (S.K.); @UjjRam (U.R.)

Psychiatr Clin N Am 42 (2019) 555–562
https://doi.org/10.1016/j.psc.2019.08.010
0193-953X/19/© 2019 Elsevier Inc. All rights reserved.

and in inner-city communities.[3] There are approximately 8200 practicing child and adolescent psychiatrists in the United States,[4] and more than 15 million youth in need of the special expertise of a child and adolescent psychiatrist.[5]

Telepsychiatry, the use of videoconferencing to provide psychiatric evaluation, consultation, supervision, education, and treatment, has potential benefits on both ends of the connection. Studies demonstrate that the clinical outcomes of care delivered via telepsychiatry are comparable to that of in-person care.[6] In some cases, care provided by telepsychiatry may be better than in person. Patients with certain diagnoses, such as posttraumatic stress disorder, autism spectrum disorder, or anxiety disorders, may prefer telepsychiatry due to feelings of control, safety, and distance created by this modality.[7] Despite the increasing use of telepsychiatry for children and adolescents, formal clinician training continues to be limited.

On the patient end, telepsychiatry can address access issues in pediatric behavioral health, limit unnecessary travel, reduce school absences and parental time off from work, bring specialty care to local communities, and improve outcomes by reducing delays in diagnosis and treatment. Children have grown up around technology and are comfortable seeing their doctor by video. Additionally, children and families in smaller, rural communities may be more willing to seek psychiatric care at a distance due to enhanced feelings of confidentiality, because it is less likely that they will run into their telepsychiatrist, who may be physically located hundreds of miles away from them.

On the practitioner end, telemedicine, including telepsychiatry, can enhance physician satisfaction with the ability to reach populations that are otherwise unreachable, streamline clinical workflows, allow better continuity of care, facilitate collaboration among virtual care teams, allow for greater flexibility in work schedules, reduce feelings of isolation, offer conveniences such as eliminating the need to commute to an office or between sites, and improve the health and well-being of physicians. When done right, the use of technology in medicine can help mitigate physician burnout. These benefits increase the likelihood of recruiting and retaining child and adolescent psychiatrists.

To ensure successful implementation and sustainability of telepsychiatry, education and training are important not only for psychiatrists but also for the entire team of health care professionals who are actively involved with the practice of telepsychiatry, including telepresenters, nurses, medical assistants, social workers, psychologists, medical students, and postgraduate trainees. Patients and guardians also should be provided with information on telepsychiatry and given the opportunity to ask questions about the care they will receive through this modality.

This article reviews the current literature on telepsychiatry education and training, provides resources including best practices and guidelines, provides an overview of considerations unique to the practice of telepsychiatry with children and adolescents, and discusses future directions to advance education and training in child and adolescent telepsychiatry.

REVIEW OF THE LITERATURE ON TELEPSYCHIATRY EDUCATION AND TRAINING

Limited literature exists on telepsychiatry education and training and the vast majority does not address considerations unique to practicing telepsychiatry with children and adolescents. Furthermore, the main focus of the evidence base is on postgraduate medical education without addressing education and training for actively practicing child and adolescent psychiatrists, who would also benefit significantly from access to reliable resources to help guide their telemedicine practice. Psychiatrists may be resistant to integrating telepsychiatry into their practice without relevant education, clinical experience, and exposure to the technology.

A majority of current medical students and postgraduate trainees are digital natives who are comfortable with technology and consider it to be an integral and necessary part of their lives. Despite the rapid expansion of technology in health care, most medical schools do not include telemedicine education and training as a required part of their curriculum. The integration of telemedicine-based lessons, ethics case studies, clinical rotations, and teleassessments offer great value for medical schools and their students.[8] Because psychiatry is one of the most common uses of telemedicine, telepsychiatry often is the first clinical exposure medical students have to telemedicine at academic medical centers. This uniquely positions our field to lead telemedicine education and training. Early training in and exposure to the use of innovative technology in medicine may help recruit medical students into child and adolescent psychiatry.

Currently, the Accreditation Council for Graduate Medical Education (ACGME), the accrediting body for psychiatry residency programs in the United States, does not require telepsychiatry training in psychiatry residencies.[9] The American Academy of Child and Adolescent Psychiatry (AACAP) and the American Psychiatric Association (APA) strongly support the inclusion of telepsychiatry education and training into graduate medical education.

A survey of psychiatry residency programs across the United States found that few programs offered a curriculum in telepsychiatry and most programs reported an interest in a sample curriculum.[10]

A literature review on telepsychiatry in graduate medical education identified 20 publications describing training psychiatry residents in telepsychiatry.[11] The majority of the literature was primarily descriptive, and the investigators concluded that a more evidence-based approach to telepsychiatry training is needed, including an assessment of residents' learning needs, use of multiple learning modalities, and evaluations of educational curricula.

Crawford and colleagues[12] used an assessment of resident learning needs to identify specific skills required for the practice of effective telepsychiatry and to provide an evidence base to guide the development of telepsychiatry curricula in postgraduate psychiatry training. The specific domains of competency identified were technical skills; assessment skills; relational skills and communication; collaborative and interprofessional skills; administrative skills; medicolegal skills; community psychiatry and community-specific knowledge; cultural psychiatry skills, including knowledge of indigenous cultures; and knowledge of health systems. Hilty and colleagues[13] proposed a framework for telepsychiatric training and e-health for trainees and clinicians, with competencies organized using the ACGME framework.

More data are needed on what core skills should be required for telepsychiatry training. To date, there are no published studies assessing telepsychiatry education and curriculum development in child and adolescent psychiatry fellowship programs in the United States.

TELEHEALTH FOR EDUCATION, CONSULTATION, AND MENTORING IN CHILD PSYCHIATRY

The benefits of telehealth extend beyond direct patient care. Videoconferencing can be used to provide telesupervision to medical trainees across a wide variety of settings and specialties, including child and adolescent psychiatry, particularly in rural and other underserved areas in the United States and internationally with limited access to local supervision.

Project Extension for Community Healthcare Outcomes (ECHO) uses telehealth technology to provide education, consultation and mentoring. It was originally established at the University of New Mexico to provide education to primary care providers (PCPs) on the management of hepatitis C. In the past decade, the model has expanded across a variety of specialties, including child and adolescent psychiatry, to provide didactic training and case-based interactive consultation to PCPs and allied health professionals. This model has been shown effective in improving patient outcomes and provider knowledge.[14]

Project ECHO is a case-based, interactive, learning collaborative model with a hub-and-spoke structure. It is designed to reduce access-to-care barriers for populations in underserved communities by using telehealth technologies to link a centrally located multidisciplinary team of specialists at a hub with PCPs in spoke communities. The hub team in psychiatry typically includes a psychiatrist, psychologist, clinical pharmacist, social worker, information technology support specialist, and program coordinator. Some hub teams may include a PCP, parent, and/or teacher to include their perspectives. The hub team specialists do not provide direct patient care to patients at spoke sites; they serve as a resource for PCPs. The facilitated discussion typically includes diagnostic guidance, suggestions for further evaluation and psychosocial support, and nonpharmacologic and pharmacologic treatment. Academic programs serving as hubs often use the program to train their psychiatry trainees in teleconsultation skills.

The Project ECHO model has been successfully used for general psychiatry as well as specialty areas, such as child and adolescent psychiatry, autism, addiction, and systems of care models like collaborative care.

Project ECHO can be used for professional development using the current criteria of continued professional development: participation, satisfaction, learning, competence, performance, patient, and community health. The model also aligns with current best practice recommendations for continued medical education.[15]

SPECIAL CONSIDERATIONS FOR TELEPSYCHIATRY WITH CHILDREN AND ADOLESCENTS

Children and adolescents in the digital age are accustomed to being connected through the use of electronics, such as social media, video games, and interactive videoconferencing applications on mobile devices (eg, FaceTime). Pediatric outcomes studies indicate that adolescents are more comfortable with telepsychiatry and treatment outcomes are comparable to in-person visits.[16,17] It is important for psychiatrists to effectively translate basic tenets of in-person interactions to psychiatric assessments conducted via telepsychiatry.

Telepsychiatry with children requires intentional actions to overcome the physical separation. In order to engage and instantly build rapport with a child, a psychiatrist can comment on curious actions, such as children making faces at the camera while watching their own image in a picture-in-picture view, or comment on children's clothing, toys, or objects they are carrying. In addition to reinforcing that a child is visible to the psychiatrist, this provides an opportunity to discuss the novel experience of a video visit before addressing clinical matters. When children are moving around due to hyperactivity, exploratory behaviors, agitation, or other reasons, however, it is important to ensure that they are in the camera frame for uninterrupted observation. Using a remotely controlled, pan-tilt-zoom camera, therefore, may be preferred in telepsychiatry with children over the integrated, stationary cameras used with adults or older adolescents. For younger children, parents can have children sit on their laps during the session if needed. For older adolescents with a parent or other individuals present, the camera may need appropriate adjustment to accommodate 2 or more individuals in the frame. Involving the adolescent and their family in this process of setting up can foster a sense of engagement and make the interaction collaborative from the beginning of the session.

Appropriate lighting and nondistracting surroundings are essential for reliable observation and assessment of any involuntary motor movements, facial expression, and subtleties of affect. Ample, indirect lighting and a clutter-free background on both ends of the connection are key for best viewing. These technical aspects of the camera and lighting assist in enhancing the quality and comfort of telepsychiatry sessions. Educators can teach these rapport-building technical considerations to residents and child and adolescent psychiatry fellows conducting telepsychiatry. Simulations using camera recordings of trainees during mock telepsychiatry sessions can serve as an excellent tool for practicing these technical aspects and skills.

Nonverbal communication plays a crucial role in creating an authentic experience through expression of empathy, professionalism, and therapeutic intentions. This is especially important when typical physical interactions like shaking hands have to be replaced by gestures on screen. With children and adolescents as the primary audience, the psychiatrist must ensure good eye contact and communicate with an exaggerated tone of voice, facial expressions, and energetic hand gestures. The psychiatrist should use appropriate camera placement to convey natural eye contact. Leaning forward can express empathy and leaning back can show interest in hearing more. Using high fives or thumbs-up on camera with youth also serve as good alternatives for verbal encouragers like "good job" and can help share more information. It is important to identify and practice nonverbal gestures, including facial expressions on camera in advance to ensure that those are visible in the camera frame during telepsychiatry sessions. Educators and supervisors can teach the basic tenets of being an empathetic listener through a deliberate emphasis on nonverbal communication in telepsychiatry.

Training in child and adolescent telepsychiatry includes staying up-to-date on the constantly evolving reimbursement, legal and regulatory environment, and new models of delivery. Key administrative, ethical, and clinical aspects, including emergency management, also must be learned.

OTHER TECHNOLOGIES

Apart from the traditional live, interactive, audio-video communication, other forms of technology also are becoming mainstream in health care; these include mobile technology integrated in phones, wearable devices, and standalone remote devices, collectively referred to as mHealth. With more than 70% of teens connected to the Internet and mobile devices, these tools are becoming important sources of data collection as well as interventions through Web-based and app-based platforms. More recently, artificial intelligence has been used to develop modalities using mobile text or conversational agents (chatbots) for cognitive-behavioral therapy interventions. The literature on these applications of technology, however, is still emerging. Educators should consider using technology curricula to better equip child and adolescent psychiatry trainees to understand the current landscape, provide guidance on how to evaluate these technologies, provide an overview of current research on feasibility and outcomes, and discuss different digital tools that can be utilized in daily practice for assessment, patient communication, treatment, and monitoring of health outcomes.[18]

PEDIATRIC TELEPSYCHIATRY EDUCATION AND TRAINING RESOURCES

Some academic medical centers provide formal orientation, education, and training in telepsychiatry to their postgraduate trainees and/or faculty; however, there is great variability in the breadth and quality of educational content, training, and clinical exposure. Large health care systems, such as the Department of Veterans Affairs and the Department of Defense, also provide telepsychiatry orientation and training to their staff.

Individual psychiatrists without access to such resources may obtain education by review of relevant scientific literature and through telepsychiatry presentations or workshops online or in-person, such as those offered through the AACAP, APA, and the American Telemedicine Association (ATA). There is no formal, nationally recognized certification in telepsychiatry. Some psychiatrists start providing clinical telepsychiatry services without baseline education or training and learn through clinical experience and consultation with colleagues.

The 2017 AACAP "Clinical Update: Telepsychiatry with Children and Adolescents"[19] reviews the use of telepsychiatry to deliver psychiatric, mental health, and care coordination services to youth across settings as direct service and in collaboration with other clinicians. The update presents procedures for conducting telepsychiatry services and optimizing the clinical experience.

The AACAP, in partnership with the APA, developed an online Child and Adolescent Telepsychiatry Toolkit[20] in 2019 to address issues unique to practicing telepsychiatry with children and adolescents. The toolkit consists of a series of video series that cover topics in telepsychiatry related to the history, training, practice and clinical issues, reimbursement, and legal issues from leading child and adolescent psychiatrists. This toolkit was developed to complement the APA's Telepsychiatry Toolkit by adding pediatric-specific considerations.

The 2017 ATA "Practice Guidelines for Telemental Health with Children and Adolescents"[21] provides a clinical guideline for the delivery of child and adolescent mental health and behavioral services by a licensed health care provider through real-time videoconferencing.

The APA and ATA released the "Best Practices in Videoconferencing-Based Telemental Health" guide[22] in 2018 to assist practitioners in providing effective and safe medical care founded on expert consensus, research evidence, available resources, and patient needs.

The telepsychiatry committees of the AACAP and ATA regularly provide up-to-date resources on telepsychiatry. **Table 1** summarizes key online resources for pediatric telepsychiatry.

FUTURE DIRECTIONS

This article provides an overview of the current literature on telepsychiatry education and training and preliminary guidance on developing education and training resources specific to pediatric telepsychiatry. Additional research is needed to assess the current state of telepsychiatry education and training in child and adolescent psychiatry fellowship programs. Future opportunities include developing an evidence-based pediatric telepsychiatry curriculum for trainees and practicing child and adolescent psychiatrists. Ongoing efforts are under way in the development of a curriculum in pediatric telebehavioral health to improve training nationally and address workforce shortages and geographic maldistribution. Future educational initiatives should address training not only for child psychiatrists but also for the entire multidisciplinary team of health care professionals who will be actively involved with the practice of

Table 1
Pediatric telepsychiatry resources and useful Web sites

Resource	Web Site
AACAP Telepsychiatry Resource Page	https://www.aacap.org/AACAP/Clinical_Practice_Center/Business_of_Practice/Telepsychiatry/Telepsych_Home.aspx
APA Telepsychiatry Toolkit	https://www.psychiatry.org/psychiatrists/practice/telepsychiatry/toolkit
Joint AACAP-APA Child and Adolescent Telepsychiatry Toolkit	https://www.psychiatry.org/psychiatrists/practice/telepsychiatry/toolkit/child-adolescent
Center for Telehealth and e-Health Law	https://ctel.org/
Center for Connected Health Policy	https://www.cchpca.org/
National Consortium of Telehealth Resource Centers	https://www.telehealthresourcecenter.org/
ATA	https://www.americantelemed.org/

All Web sites were accessed May 15, 2019.

telepsychiatry, including telepresenters, nurses, medical assistants, social workers, psychologists, and medical students.

ACKNOWLEDGMENT

A special thanks to the AACAP Telepsychiatry Committee, and Drs. Kathleen Myers, Sandra DeJong, and David Pruitt.

REFERENCES

1. Williams NJ, Scott L, Aarons GA. Prevalence of serious emotional disturbance among U.S. children: a meta-analysis. Psychiatr Serv 2018;69(1):32–40.
2. Jones PB. Adult mental health disorders and their age at onset. Br J Psychiatry Suppl 2013;54:s5–10.
3. Flaum M. Telemental health as a solution to the widening gap between supply and demand for mental health services. In: Myers K, Turvey C, editors. Telemental health: clinical, technical and administrative foundation for evidence-based practice. London: Elsevier Insights; 2013. p. 11–25.
4. American Medical Association. Physician masterfile. 2017. Available at: https://www.ama-assn.org/practice-management/masterfile/ama-physician-masterfile. Accessed March 1, 2019.
5. AACAP resources for primary care: workforce issues. Available at: https://www.aacap.org/aacap/resources_for_primary_care/Workforce_Issues.aspx. Accessed April 15, 2019.
6. O'Reilly R, Bishop J, Maddox K, et al. Is telepsychiatry equivalent to face-to-face psychiatry? Results from a randomized controlled equivalence trial. Psychiatr Serv 2007;58(6):836–43.
7. Shore JH, Savin DM, Novins D, et al. Cultural aspects of telepsychiatry. J Telemed Telecare 2006;12(3):116–21.
8. Waseh S, Dicker AP. Telemedicine training in undergraduate medical education: mixed-methods review. JMIR Med Educ 2019;5(1):e12515.
9. Accreditation Council for Graduate Medical Education (ACGME). Program requirements for graduate medical education in psychiatry 2017. Available at: https://www.

acgme.org/Portals/0/PFAssets/ProgramRequirements/400_psychiatry_2017-07-01. pdf. Accessed April 15, 2019.

10. Hoffman P, Kane JM. Telepsychiatry education and curriculum development in residency training. Acad Psychiatry 2015;39(1):108–9.

11. Sunderji N, Crawford A, Jovanovic M. Telepsychiatry in graduate medical education: a narrative review. Acad Psychiatry 2015;39(1):55–62.

12. Crawford A, Sunderji N, Lopez J, et al. Defining competencies for the practice of telepsychiatry through an assessment of resident learning needs. BMC Med Educ 2016;16:28.

13. Hilty DM, Crawford A, Teshima J, et al. A framework for telepsychiatric training and e-health: competency-based education, evaluation and implications. Int Rev Psychiatry 2015;27(6):569–92.

14. Zhou C, Crawford A, Serhal E, et al. The impact of project ECHO on participant and patient outcomes: a systematic review. Acad Med 2016;91(10):1439–61.

15. Arora S, Kalishman SG, Thornton KA, et al. Project ECHO: a telementoring network model for continuing professional development. J Contin Educ Health Prof 2017;37(4):239–44.

16. Elford R, White H, Bowering R, et al. A randomized, controlled trial of child psychiatric assessments conducted using videoconferencing. J Telemed Telecare 2000;6(2):73–82.

17. Myers K, Vander Stoep A, McCarty C, et al. Child and adolescent telepsychiatry: Variations in utilization, referral patterns and practice trends. J Telemed Telecare 2010;16:128.

18. Gipson SY-MT, Kim JW, Shin AL, et al. Teaching child and adolescent psychiatry in the twenty-first century. Child Adolesc Psychiatr Clin N Am 2017;26(1):93–103.

19. American Academy of Child and Adolescent Psychiatry (AACAP) Committee on Telepsychiatry and AACAP Committee on Quality Issues. Clinical update: telepsychiatry with children and adolescents. J Am Acad Child Adolesc Psychiatry 2017;56(10):875–93.

20. AACAP-APA child and adolescent telepsychiatry toolkit. 2019. Available at: https://www.psychiatry.org/psychiatrists/practice/telepsychiatry/toolkit/child-adolescent. Accessed April 15, 2019.

21. Myers K, Nelson EL, Rabinowitz T, et al. American telemedicine association practice guidelines for telemental health with children and adolescents. Telemed J E Health 2017;23(10):779–804.

22. Shore JH, Yellowlees P, Caudill R, et al. Best practices in videoconferencing-based telemental health April 2018. Telemed J E Health 2018;24(11):827–32.

Personalized Implementation of Video Telehealth

Jan A. Lindsay, PhD[a,b,c,*], Stephanie C. Day, PhD[a,c],
Amber B. Amspoker, PhD[b,c], Terri L. Fletcher, PhD[a,b,c],
Julianna Hogan, PhD[a,b,c], Giselle Day, MPH[a,b], Ashley Helm, MA[a,b],
Melinda A. Stanley, PhD[c], Lindsey A. Martin, PhD[b,c]

KEYWORDS

- Telemedicine • Veterans • Mental health • Implementation
- Health services research • Delivery of health care

KEY POINTS

- Implementing video telehealth to home (VTH) within large medical systems relies heavily on a flexible implementation strategy that involves external and internal facilitation.
- Providing mental health treatment via VTH allows patients and providers to overcome many barriers to treatment and provides patients greater choice about when and where they receive their care.
- Implementing a sustainable VTH program should start small by identifying dedicated clinical champions and celebrating early successes.
- Measuring multiple variables to evaluate the breadth and depth of VTH delivery and the implementation strategy can increase impact.

The authors report no financial conflicts of interest.
This work was supported by a grant from the VA Office of Rural Health, Salt Lake City Resource Center and partly supported by the use of facilities and resources of the Houston VA HSR&D Center for Innovations in Quality, Effectiveness and Safety (CIN13-413) and the VA South Central Mental Illness Research, Education and Clinical Center. The opinions expressed are those of the authors and not necessarily those of the Department of Veterans Affairs, the US government, or Baylor College of Medicine.
[a] VA South Central Mental Illness Research, Education and Clinical Center (a virtual center);
[b] Houston VA HSR&D Center for Innovations in Quality, Effectiveness and Safety, Michael E. DeBakey VA Medical Center (MEDVAMC152), 2002 Holcombe Boulevard, Houston, TX 77030, USA; [c] Department of Psychiatry and Behavioral Sciences, Baylor College of Medicine, One Baylor Plaza, Houston, TX 77030, USA
* Corresponding author. Houston VA HSR&D Center for Innovations in Quality, Effectiveness and Safety, Michael E. DeBakey Veterans Affairs Medical Center, (MEDVAMC 152), 2002 Holcombe Blvd., Houston, TX 77030.
E-mail address: Jan.Lindsay2@va.gov

Psychiatr Clin N Am 42 (2019) 563–574
https://doi.org/10.1016/j.psc.2019.08.001
0193-953X/19/Published by Elsevier Inc.

psych.theclinics.com

INTRODUCTION

Notable logistical, financial, and stigma-related barriers to engaging in and being retained in mental health (MH) care exist. Those who seek MH care often have difficulty accessing specialty or evidence-based treatment and may not receive an adequate dose to address their MH issues.[1,2] Telehealth programs for MH care, specifically, clinical videoconferencing, have not reached their potential in increasing access to care, largely due to system complexities in implementation,[3-5] including technical difficulties for support staff and challenges of integration into clinical workflow.[6] Although patient satisfaction with telehealth programs is high, provider adoption is slow. For example, providers have concerns over the impact of video technology on the provider-patient relationship, logistical (eg, scheduling) issues, and complexities associated with the technology.[6-9] Implementation approaches with concrete steps and guidance are needed to fully leverage telehealth technology for widespread use.

Initially, MH telehealth in the Veterans Health Administration (VHA) was conducted clinic-to-clinic, allowing providers at a large facility to remotely deliver care to patients in another clinic location. However, this approach did not fully address logistical, financial, and transportation barriers, given the patients still had to travel to the community clinic. Video telehealth to home (VTH) is another form of telehealth that enables patients to connect with MH provider directly from home or another convenient, private location of their choice (**Fig. 1**). VTH can increase access to care and retention in MH treatment and is as effective as in-person care.[10]

Developing telehealth programs within a hospital or clinic system has often involved creating silos (ie, providers within a medical center who deliver care only via telehealth) or telehealth centers (ie, providers in a remote/distant location who use telehealth delivery to address gaps or personnel shortages). These models allow providers to become extremely proficient in telehealth delivery of care and overcome provider shortage concerns in underserved areas by allowing providers in one geographic region to provide care to patients in another. However, silo and telehealth center models eliminate the possibility of meeting with patients in person when necessary or when preferred by patients because providers often are in geographically distant locations and/or do not have access to traditional office space.

Integrated models of VTH maximize patient choice by offering the option to meet with providers either in person or virtually, as preferred. When many providers across a clinic or health care system are trained to deliver care via VTH as one aspect of their clinical role, patients and providers can collaboratively determine the mode of delivery

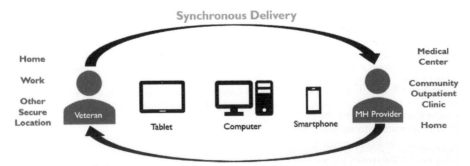

Fig. 1. VA video connect technology.

(eg, all in-person, all VTH, a combination of in-person and VTH) that is most convenient and clinically appropriate. For example, a patient with transportation or childcare barriers can request a VTH appointment instead of canceling. Similarly, a provider can ask a patient who is decompensating to come in person to the next appointment.

Despite notable benefits of VTH for patient care and clinical practice and high levels of patient satisfaction,[11–14] VTH utilization in the VHA has not expanded as quickly as expected or desired, demonstrating a need for effective and replicable implementation approaches that increase uptake of VTH among providers and clinics. This article describes a clinical demonstration project for which the authors developed a specific implementation approach, Personalized Implementation for Video Telehealth (PIVOT), to increase adoption of VTH across a large, urban VA Medical Center (VAMC). Development of PIVOT for implementation of VTH was anchored in Implementation Facilitation,[15] a strategy responsive to contextual factors that promotes the uptake of innovations in health care settings through activities, including stakeholder engagement, innovation messaging, and technical support, among others.[15–18] The adaptive nature of this approach allows responsiveness to technological and contextual changes, both nationally and locally, that affect VTH implementation.

The authors first provide historical context about the use of VTH in the VHA Health Care System. Thereafter, they describe the development and application of PIVOT, a strategy that allowed them to maximize patient choice and incorporate VTH into general practice, compared with a silo or telehealth center approach. They review how the use of PIVOT helps to engage health-system leadership and key stakeholders and identify Internal Facilitators and Clinical Champions to promote change. The authors describe their implementation process and strategies used to meet implementation goals, with a special focus on formative and summative outcomes that demonstrate how PIVOT led to overall satisfaction and sustained growth of VTH at this VAMC. They also offer recommendations for implementing a VTH program using the PIVOT strategy.

VIDEO TELEHEALTH TO HOME IN THE VA: HISTORICAL OVERVIEW

Several developments over the past 5 years within the VHA expanded the reach of telehealth and significantly changed the VTH technology platform (**Table 1**).

PERSONALIZED IMPLEMENTATION OF VIDEO TELEHEALTH

The PIVOT approach (**Fig. 2**) developed as the authors sought to fully integrate VTH into existing MH clinics over 5 years (FY14 through FY18) at the Houston VAMC. The Houston project was the next iteration that built on a smaller-scale implementation effort in Jackson, MS, which used a similar approach but focused solely on the delivery of evidence-based psychotherapies to increase access to rural patients.[19] The Houston VAMC serves approximately 130,000 Veterans at its main campus and network of 11 community clinics. To maximize patient choice, VTH was incorporated into general practice across multiple MH clinics (rather than training specific providers to deliver only VTH) as one option for care delivery, improving continuity of care and increasing the likelihood that VTH would be sustained and integrated into routine clinical care.

Evolving technological innovations and VHA priorities necessitated a nimble implementation approach to allow real-time communication about technology and policy changes to MH leadership and providers at the Houston VAMC. The PIVOT approach can be adapted to address different health-system contexts and specific innovations. It uses expert External Facilitators (licensed clinicians with expertise in implementation

Table 1
Historical developments of video telehealth to home within the VHA system

Year	Developments in VA	Details
2013	Approval to provide MH via VTH	Cumbersome for patients and providers (software-based, required usernames & passwords to connect)
2017	Expansion of telehealth	Support for telehealth services across state lines (no official policy) Focus on Veterans in remote or rural areas
2017	National introduction of VA Video Connect platform	More user friendly (web-based program, eliminates usernames and passwords); allows delivery of MH care via personal computer, tablet or smartphone, with VHA providing device if necessary Mandate that >5% Veterans will receive some care through telehealth to home or mobile device in FY18
2018	Expansion of telehealth services into the home and other non-VA settings	Official policy approving anywhere-to-anywhere delivery All telehealth services within VHA under umbrella of federal supremacy Mandate that 100% of MH providers be trained in VTH by end of FY20

science and telehealth technology); Internal Facilitators (individuals with knowledge of the hospital system and existing relationships with providers who are empowered to be local VTH point of contact); and Clinical Champions (providers located in satellite community or specialty MH clinics who inform colleagues and patients about VTH) to increase uptake of VTH throughout a medical system. External Facilitators simultaneously gather and coalesce information while training, supporting, and empowering on-site Internal Facilitators to implement and sustain VTH. The External Facilitators' credentials and expertise maximize their credibility as the authors engage key stakeholders in implementing VTH.

The first step of PIVOT is an initial meeting with External Facilitators, health-system leadership, and key stakeholders (eg, information technology, MH leadership, site telehealth lead) to discuss nationally established, system-wide implementation goals; present evidence for VTH; and consult about where to initiate implementation efforts. External Facilitators then identify on-site Internal Facilitators, often community or specialty clinic supervisors, with knowledge of the local system, influence, and existing relationships with providers. The focus on long-term sustainability necessitates training Internal Facilitators in VTH delivery and empowering each to become a local VTH expert, with support from External Facilitators. External Facilitators also help Internal Facilitators identify Clinical Champion providers across clinics and disciplines (eg, psychiatry, psychology, social work, masters-level counselors) to maximize uptake. Ideally, one Clinical Champion is identified in each satellite community or specialty MH (ie, posttraumatic stress disorder [PTSD], General MH, Women's Health, Substance Dependence Treatment, Primary Care MH Integration) clinic where VTH implementation will occur. External Facilitators train Clinical Champions in VTH delivery, then mentor and empower Internal Facilitators to provide support and guidance to ensure consistent, positive VTH messaging. External Facilitators continue to provide Internal Facilitators with support, resources (ie, note templates, emergency guidance), and troubleshooting to help them create and sustain a VTH program.

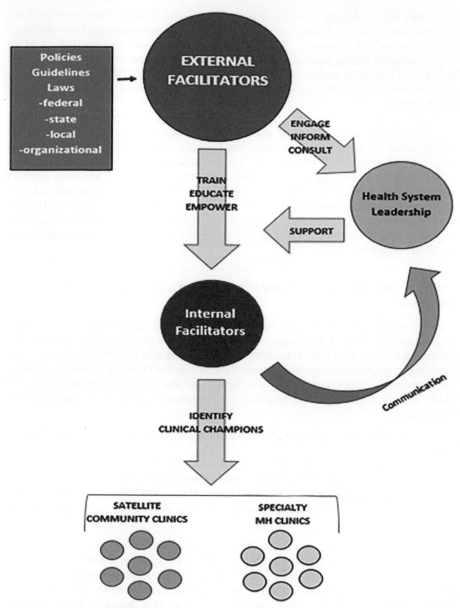

Fig. 2. Overview of PIVOT approach.

Throughout the implementation process, External Facilitators review and compile multilevel (federal, state, local, organizational) best practices, ethical guidelines, laws, and mandates concerning VTH delivery, technology, and compensation. During early stages of implementation, External Facilitators are responsible for communicating the latest developments in VTH policy to site leadership and Internal Facilitators. In preparation for sustainability, Internal Facilitators are encouraged to take an active role in expanding and sustaining the innovation, with guidance from External Facilitators on how to access information directly and to communicate with site leadership about relevant changes. This process helps External Facilitators shift responsibilities to Internal Facilitators and allows greater communication between Internal Facilitators and leadership. The transition to sustainment can be thought of as titrating external efforts down and placing a greater emphasis on engagement at the local level. During the sustainment phase, the role of External Facilitators transforms to a consultative role, with responsibility for active problem-solving shifting to Internal Facilitators.

The initial focus on empowering early adopter clinical champions, who identified themselves as being enthusiastic about the VTH-delivery modality, enabled us to quickly enter the system and demonstrate success, before VHA instituted national mandates. However, truly integrated implementation of VTH, or any innovation, requires more than engagement of a few early adopters. PIVOT involves ongoing communication with MH providers, clinic leadership, site leadership, and national telehealth to clarify expectations and shift the system's perceptions about VTH. The authors' iterative approach provided ongoing opportunities to assess the benefits of VTH and communicate them back to MH providers, thus increasing motivation and sustained adoption.

OUTCOME EVALUATION OF PERSONALIZED IMPLEMENTATION FOR VIDEO TELEHEALTH

Outcome evaluation of VTH implementation included both quantitative and qualitative data collection. To test the impact of this implementation approach, the authors compared rates of VTH use in Houston VAMC and affiliated community clinics to national VHA data, which were collected via the VHA Support Service Center Capital Assets Databases. They chose to examine the prevalence of 5 outcomes at the Houston VAMC and national levels to capture both the breadth and depth of a sustainable telehealth clinic:

1. Linear change in number of patients receiving MH services via VTH from FY13 to FY18,
2. Linear change in number of VTH visits from FY13 to FY18,
3. Number of MH providers delivering services via VTH in FY18,
4. Number of unique specialty-care MH clinics offering VTH services in FY18, and
5. Number of community clinics active in delivering VTH at any point from FY14 to FY18.

As nationwide data were positively skewed (all Shapiro-Wilks $Ps < 0.0001$), five 1-sample median (Sign) tests were used to compare Houston with the median nationwide value on each outcome. Sites identified by VHA as designated telemental health hubs ($n = 11$) were excluded from analyses because they received temporary dedicated funding for staff to deliver telehealth, as part of a larger national initiative. **Table 2** presents demographic data for patients who received VTH in Houston between FY14 and FY18.

Change in the number of unique patients receiving VTH and the number of VTH visits for the Houston VAMC and nationwide from FY14 to FY18 are presented in **Figs. 3** and **4**. Houston showed a significantly greater increase in the number of unique Veterans receiving VTH (linear slope = 59.71) and the number of VTH encounters (linear slope = 248.91) than other VAMCs (median slopes of 9.51 and 38.11, respectively), Sign Test M = −58.5 and −55.5, respectively, both $Ps < 0.0001$. In fact, the increase in the number of patients receiving VTH and VTH visits was 6.3 and 6.5 times (respectively) greater for Houston relative to median national improvement.

Table 2
Demographic data for the patients who received VTH in Houston between FY14 and FY18 (N = 619)

	N (%)
Male	405 (65.43%)
Age (y)	
20–29	83 (13.41%)
30–39	229 (37.00%)
40–49	128 (20.68%)
50–59	101 (16.32%)
60–69	51 (8.24%)
70–79	24 (3.88%)
80–89	3 (0.48%)
Urban Residence	491 (79.32%)
OEF/OIF/OND[a]	
Yes	212 (34.25%)
No/Unknown	407 (65.75%)

[a] Veterans returning from the recent conflicts in Iraq and Afghanistan.

Furthermore, Houston had 47 MH providers who provided VTH in FY18, which was significantly greater (3.92 times greater) than the national median (ie, 12 providers), Sign Test M = −58.5, $P<0.0001$. Depth of VTH integration was evidenced by a significantly greater number of unique specialty MH clinics offering VTH in Houston in FY18 (n = 7) and a greater number of community clinics active in delivering VTH at any point from FY14 to FY18 (n = 7), numbers that were significantly greater (3.5 and 7 times greater, respectively) than the national median of 2 and 1 (respectively), Sign Test M = −61 and −55.5, respectively, both $Ps < 0.0001$.

To inform ongoing implementation efforts, the authors gathered qualitative feedback from VTH providers about their experiences with this modality. Providers noted how VTH enabled patients to receive care for low-incidence MH issues (ie, obsessive-compulsive disorder), more effectively treated certain disorders (ie, ability to see home environment of patients with hoarding; patients with agoraphobia do not need to resolve anxiety to receive care), and reach patients who would otherwise not engage in care due to issues or conditions that make coming to a VAMC or community clinic difficult (ie, PTSD, military sexual trauma, and chronic pain or physical disability).

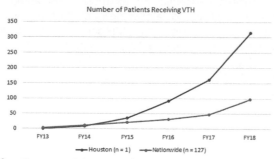

Fig. 3. Number of patients receiving VTH from FY13 to FY18 at the Houston VAMC and Nationwide.

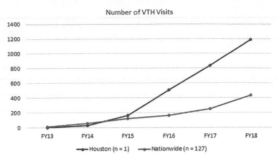

Fig. 4. Number of unique VTH visits from FY13 to FY18 at the MEDVAMC and Nationwide.

Providers also highlighted logistical and clinical concerns (eg, handling emergency situations over video, whether providing care into the home was "enabling" avoidant behavior) that the authors were able to preemptively address with newly trained VTH providers. One notable contextual change that providers described as affecting implementation efforts was Hurricane Harvey. See sidebar for additional information describing conditions in Houston during part of this project. The authors believe that these conditions contributed, in part, to their successful outcome by illustrating the usefulness of VTH, especially in times of crisis/natural disaster.

The authors conducted qualitative interviews with a representative, diverse sample of Veterans (n = 30) who had at least 3 MH visits via VTH to evaluate Veteran satisfaction with VTH. Veterans reported liking the convenience of VTH, as well as the comfort and privacy of receiving MH care at home. Most patients (83.3%) reported at least one barrier to engaging in MH treatment, with anxiety about leaving home being the most commonly identified barrier to accessing in-person care at a VAMC or affiliated clinic (67%). Distance/travel time (63%), taking time off work (50%), lack of comfort at VA (43%), and physical limitations (37%) were reported as other notable barriers.

RECOMMENDATIONS FOR IMPLEMENTING A VIDEO TELEHEALTH TO HOME PROGRAM

During the demonstration project, the authors identified several recommendations for implementing VTH. **Table 3** presents an overview and expansion of PIVOT recommendations to illustrate how this personalized implementation strategy might be effectively adapted for use outside VHA medical centers.

Engage Leadership Early and Often

When implementing VTH, either in a VA or non-VA setting, engaging leadership early in the implementation process is essential. For example, in the authors' demonstration project, engaging the telehealth coordinator at the local site, the clinic supervisor where implementation is taking place, and the lead of MH services at the facility promoted uptake. Leadership buy-in is critical to highlighting the importance of VTH implementation to providers at the facility, including the investment of resources to support implementation and the identification of incentives to promote adoption (eg, provider-level: flexible work schedule, telework options; clinic-level: conserves valuable resources such as space). Regularly communicating implementation progress and outcome metrics (see last point below) helps to foster ongoing leadership engagement.

Make Facilitation Key

External facilitation is key for developing successful, sustainable VTH programs again with likely relevance to both VA and non-VA systems. Based on the authors'

Table 3
Application of Personalized Implementation for Video Telehealth

Recommendation	Considerations & Adaptations
Engage leadership early and often	• Obtain leadership buy-in and investment of resources • Establish ongoing communication to inform leadership on implementation progress/changes • Provide periodic feedback on outcome metrics from available data sources • Identify incentives to motivate provider adoption of VTH
Make facilitation key	• External facilitators provide expertise in innovation, engage leadership, and track policy changes • Local site internal facilitators need (1) protected time to support implementation and (2) training in facilitation and the clinical innovation
Start small to optimize success	• Engage stakeholders at every level of the organization • Collaboratively set realistic implementation goals • Early adopter providers and/or clinics to pilot the implementation plan • Identify motivating aspects/elements to boost provider and leadership adoption (eg, patient success stories; reduced no-shows)
Ensure flexibility	• Each site has unique barriers/facilitators • Adapt the implementation strategy to meet site needs • Capitalize on opportunities to illustrate the value of the innovation to ambivalent stakeholders
Assess multiple outcomes	• Identify outcome metrics of value to stakeholders • Identify persons responsible for outcome assessment • Additional outcome metrics are needed beyond those in national directives/policies • Revisit outcomes and how to measure/assess sustainability

experiences, national mandates or training requirements are insufficient to increase innovation uptake and create real practice change, particularly for complex technology-based innovations such as VTH. Using a facilitation approach such as PIVOT allows personalized assessment of the local medical system and a thorough understanding of the barriers and facilitators to implementing the innovation as well as offering external motivation, feedback about progress, and practical assistance to increase adoption. Several resources are available to support the use of external facilitation. The Agency for Healthcare Research and Quality (www.ahrq.gov), the North American Primary Care Research Group (International Conference on Practice Facilitation, www.napcrg.org), and the VA's Quality Enhancement Research Initiative (www.queri.research.va.gov) provide guidance in gaining facilitation skills to implement and sustain clinical innovations.

Start Small to Optimize Success

By starting with a "grassroots" facilitation approach, the authors were able to identify a few highly motivated providers and offer personalized "concierge" facilitation to maximize provider engagement and success. Their ability to help move providers from not only becoming trained in VTH to actively delivering care via VTH further enhanced their credibility with and buy-in from key stakeholders (eg, medical center leadership, Internal Facilitators, other potential VTH providers). Starting small also enabled them to control the message and reduce misinformation about the technology, directly addressing concerns and disseminating updates as they became available. A "grass-roots" approach can help identify early adopters and clinics within a health system where the implementation plan can be piloted and adapted to the local context.

Ensure Flexibility

Technology-based innovations, including VTH, are complicated and constantly changing. VTH involves an interrelated web of logistical, technological, and ethical considerations. In addition to advances in technology, regulations at both the national and state levels are also growing and adapting, as MH providers consider applications of novel innovations and the ethics of their safety and effectiveness. For example, medical centers must ensure their computers and internet can maintain a stable connection while adhering to national guidelines for encryption/confidentiality and documenting providers' VTH training. Each site, clinic, and provider, regardless of health system and/or clinical setting, must be assessed for readiness to change, existing infrastructure or ability to develop infrastructure, and the negotiation between national, state, and site-specific guidelines. The External Facilitators use an Implementation Checklist developed specifically for VTH that can be adapted to unique contexts, but others may choose to create their own.

Assess Multiple Outcomes to Demonstrate Impact

Frameworks for assessing the spread of new interventions have historically focused on the number of patients reached and the total number of visits. These outcomes, however, are insufficient to demonstrate fully the impact of an innovation or implementation effort. High numbers of patients or visits could reflect simply a small number of highly productive providers rather than broad success in integrating VTH care delivery throughout a clinic or site. Tracking other outcomes, including number of providers trained *and* delivering care via VTH, number of affiliated community or specialty MH clinics offering VTH, and disciplines of providers (ie, psychiatry, psychology, social work) more accurately reflects the breadth and depth of implementation. Evaluation of implementation approaches and efforts also should include qualitative data collected in both formative (ie, evaluating the project while ongoing) and summative (ie, evaluation that occurs at or toward the end of the project) phases. These kinds of data are complementary and enrich our understanding of system-level change and how to bring best practices to our patients. Assessing outcomes during implementation and feeding this information back to key stakeholders increases motivation and momentum for practice change and enables sites to respond to challenges in real time.

SUMMARY

The PIVOT approach to implementing VTH supports patient-centered health care by integrating VTH into existing clinics and offering patients the choice to see their providers in person and/or via VTH; the evaluation data indicate a marked increase in the number of patients seen via VTH and overall satisfaction with this mode of MH care delivery. Veteran feedback highlights how VTH offers convenience and meets Veterans where they are; Veteran satisfaction with VTH-delivered MH care has important implications for retaining Veterans within the VA system.

Personalizing implementation enables greater responsiveness to provider needs and can address issues/concerns in real time to prevent the spread of misinformation about telehealth delivery (eg, that VTH is not as effective as providing care in person in the clinic setting). The evaluation data show that taking this personalized approach that is flexible to the contextual issues the providers face in their individual clinic settings can have a marked increase in the overall number of providers using VTH compared with national average.

Although the authors used PIVOT to implement VTH at one VAMC, the success of their clinical demonstration project indicates viability of this approach for larger-scale dissemination of VTH both within and outside VHA. As health care rapidly shifts toward more technology-enabled care via mobile apps to help patients track their health status, patient portals to communicate with health care providers, and asynchronous web-based care, PIVOT shows promise as a flexible implementation strategy that can be adapted for any technology-based MH care innovation. In addition, PIVOT's approach of fully integrating VTH within existing clinics meets the demand for more patient-centered and patient-driven care in public health and community settings, allowing patients to receive MH care when and where they desire to best meet their access needs.

Within large health care systems such as the VHA, there is increasing emphasis on leveraging telehealth to expand access to MH treatment and offer patients more choice in how and where they receive their care. PIVOT is responsive to these priorities by creating sustainable VTH programs that modernize care delivery from medical facilities and their affiliated community outpatient clinics, growing the number of providers capable of delivering MH care via VTH to increase access to care and provide patients more choice in how their care is delivered. Essential elements of PIVOT include encouraging leadership involvement from day one, relying on facilitation to overcome challenges, letting the program grow naturally, and being flexible, and looking at the "big picture" regarding outcomes can help implementation efforts succeed where they have, perhaps, failed before. The PIVOT approach can also be adapted to implement other technology-based innovations to expand access to MH treatment.

Side Bar

In August of 2017, Houston experienced a natural disaster, Hurricane Harvey, that caused widespread devastation (eg, catastrophic flooding, power outages, property damage). Thousands of individuals stayed in emergency shelters after being displaced from their homes and were without transportation (ie, personal cars were flooded, public transportation was limited). Providers relayed stories of Veterans with PTSD who were sleeping in makeshift shelters and reporting feeling distressed by the sound of search and rescue helicopters flying overhead. VTH offered a mechanism for providers and patients to connect and maintain continuity of MH treatment during this crisis. VTH delivery benefited both Veteran patients and providers who were unable to travel to the VAMC or were residing in a shelter or in an area temporarily inundated by flooding. Although Hurricane Harvey was impossible to anticipate, it offered unique motivation for previously reluctant providers to use VTH delivery to connect with their patients during the crisis and beyond.

REFERENCES

1. Olfson M, Marcus SC. National trends in outpatient psychotherapy. Am J Psychiatry 2010;167(12):1456–63.
2. Mojtabai R, Olfson M. National trends in psychotherapy by office-based psychiatrists. Arch Gen Psychiatry 2008;65:962–70.
3. Shigekawa E, Fix M, Corbett G, et al. The current state of telehealth evidence: a rapid review. Health Aff (Millwood) 2018;37(12):1975–82.

4. Kane CK, Gillis K. The use of telemedicine by physicians: Still the exception rather than the rule. Health Aff (Millwood) 2018;37(12):1923–9.
5. Ellimoottil C, An L, Moyer M, et al. Challenges and opportunities faced by large health systems implementing telehealth. Health Aff (Millwood) 2018;37(12): 1955–9.
6. Kruse CS, Krowski N, Rodriguez B, et al. Telehealth and patient satisfaction: a systematic review and narrative analysis. BMJ Open 2017;7(8):e016242.
7. Brooks E, Turvey C, Augusterfer EF. Provider barriers to telemental health: obstacles overcome, obstacles remaining. Telemed J E Health 2013;19:433–7.
8. Rees CS, Stone S. Therapeutic alliance in face-to-face versus videoconferenced psychotherapy. Prof Psychol Res Pract 2005;36:649.
9. Jameson JP, Farmer MS, Head KJ, et al. VA community mental health service providers' utilization of and attitudes toward telemental health care: the gatekeeper's perspective. J Rural Health 2011;27:425–32.
10. Fletcher TL, Hogan JB, Keegan F, et al. Recent advances in delivering mental health treatment via video to home. Curr Psychiatry Rep 2018;20(8):56.
11. Luxton DD, Pruitt LD, O'Brien K, et al. An evaluation of the feasibility and safety of a home-based telemental health treatment for posttraumatic stress in the U. S Military Telemed. J E Health 2015;21(11):1–7.
12. Campbell R, O'Gorman J, Cernovsky ZZ. Reactions of psychiatric patients to telepsychiatry. Ment Illn 2015;7(2):54–5.
13. Choi NG, Wilson NL, Sirrianni L, et al. Acceptance of home-based telehealth problem-solving therapy for depressed, low-income homebound older adults: qualitative interviews with the participants and aging-service case managers. Gerontologist 2013;54(4):704–13.
14. Gros DF, Lancaster CL, Lopez CM, et al. Treatment satisfaction of home-based telehealth versus in-person delivery of prolonged exposure for combat-related PTSD in veterans. J Telemed Telecare 2016;24(1):1–5.
15. Ritchie MJ, Dollar KM, Miller CJ, et al. Using implementation facilitation to improve care in the Veterans Health Administration (Version 2). Veterans Health Administration, Quality Enhancement Research Initiative (QUERI) for team-based behavioral health. 2017. Available at: https://www.queri.research.va.gov/tools/implementation/Facilitation-Manual.pdf. Accessed February 15, 2019.
16. Baskerville NB, Liddy C, Hogg W. Systematic review and meta-analysis of practice facilitation within primary care settings. Ann Fam Med 2012;10:63–74.
17. Kirchner JE, Ritchie MJ, Pitcock JA, et al. Outcomes of a partnered facilitation strategy to implement primary care-mental health. J Gen Intern Med 2014; 29(Suppl 4):904–12.
18. Ritchie MJ, Parker LE, Kirchner JE. Using implementation facilitation to foster clinical practice quality and adherence to evidence in challenged settings: a qualitative study. BMC Health Serv Res 2017;17:294.
19. Lindsay JA, Hudson S, Martin L, et al. Implementing video to home to increase access to evidence-based psychotherapy for rural veterans. J Technol Behav Sci 2017;2(3–4):140–8.

Clinical Lessons from Virtual House Calls in Mental Health

The Doctor Is in the House

Julianna Hogan, PhD[a,b,c,d,*], Derrecka Boykin, PhD[b,c,e],
Christopher D. Schneck, MD[f,g], Anthony H. Ecker, PhD[a,b,c,d],
Terri L. Fletcher, PhD[a,b,c,d], Jan A. Lindsay, PhD[a,b,c,d],
Jay H. Shore, MD, MPH[h]

KEYWORDS

• Video-to-home • Technology • Telehealth • Case study

Continued

Disclosure Statement: This work was funded by the Veterans Rural Health Resource Center Salt Lake City, Office of Rural Health, US Department of Veterans Affairs. The views expressed in this article are those of the authors and do not necessarily reflect the position or policy of the Department of Veterans Affairs. Visit www.ruralhealth.va.gov to learn more. This work was partly supported by the use of resources and facilities of the Houston VA HSR&D Center for Innovations in Quality, Effectiveness, and Safety (CIN13-413). The opinions expressed reflect those of the authors and not necessarily those of the Department of Veterans Affairs, the US government, or Baylor College of Medicine. This work was partly supported by National Institutes of Mental Health (R56 MH117131-01).

[a] Houston VA HSR&D Center for Innovations in Quality, Effectiveness and Safety, Michael E. DeBakey VA Medical Center (MEDVAMC152), 2002 Holcombe Boulevard, Houston, TX 77030, USA; [b] Department of Psychiatry and Behavioral Sciences, Baylor College of Medicine, One Baylor Plaza, Houston, TX 77030, USA; [c] VA South Central Mental Illness Research, Education and Clinical Center (a Virtual Center), Houston, TX, USA; [d] Department of Veterans Affairs, 2450 Holcombe Boulevard, Suite 01Y, Houston, TX 77021, USA; [e] Michael E. DeBakey VA Medical Center, 2002 Holcombe Boulevard (152), Houston, TX 77030, USA; [f] Helen and Arthur E. Johnson Depression Center, University of Colorado Hospital Infectious Disease/HIV Group Practice, 13199 East Montview Boulevard, Suite 330, Aurora, CO 80045, USA; [g] Department of Psychiatry and Family Medicine, University of Colorado School of Medicine, Anschutz Medical Campus, Aurora, CO 80045, USA; [h] Department of Psychiatry and Family Medicine, School of Medicine, Centers for American Indian and Alaska Native Health, Colorado School of Public Health, Telemedicine Helen and Arthur E. Johnson Depression Center, University of Colorado Anschutz Medical Campus, 13055 East 17th Avenue, Aurora, CO 80045, USA
* Corresponding author. Department of Veterans Affairs, 2450 Holcombe Boulevard, Suite 01Y, Houston, TX 77021.
E-mail address: Julianna.Hogan@va.gov

Psychiatr Clin N Am 42 (2019) 575–586
https://doi.org/10.1016/j.psc.2019.08.004
0193-953X/19/© 2019 Elsevier Inc. All rights reserved.

Continued

KEY POINTS

- Advances in technology and innovation have afforded greater flexibility in how, when, and where patients receive services.
- The use of video-to-home (VTH) telehealth is a patient-centered approach to clinical care that allows providers to tailor care to specific need of individual patients.
- A series of case vignettes are presented in order to help challenge provider's existing beliefs about who may be a good clinical fit for VTH.
- The authors suggest that continued education and training as well as generating or joining a community of practice will help providers achieve greater comfort and competence with VTH.

INTRODUCTION

Technology-based solutions have improved access to effective evidence-based mental health care services for many patients who may otherwise receive limited treatment, or worse, go without care.[1] Telehealth to the home, also known as video-to-home (VTH), is a delivery modality in which mental health providers connect with patients through use of a live, interactive, Web-based, video-conferencing feature via personal computers, laptops, tablets, or other similar devices. Until recently, the most common method of telehealth was clinic-to-clinic delivery, whereby a provider at 1 clinic would reach a patient physically located at a different clinic. VTH now moves the location of care from clinical settings into the patient's home or other private location. It also differs from other synchronous and asynchronous technologies, such as telephone-only services or store-and-forward (asynchronous) telehealth. Although remote delivery of care using videoconferencing is not new (eg, clinic-to-clinic telehealth services), VTH has increased the reach of care to patients who may experience considerable logistical and sociocultural barriers to care, allowing care to be delivered directly to them at home. This article highlights potential benefits and considerations for providers interested in expanding their use of VTH to engage patients who are difficult to reach or who have complex presentations.

BENEFITS OF VIDEO-TO-HOME FOR PATIENTS AND PROVIDERS

VTH is an innovative delivery method that promotes patient-centered care by giving the patient more control over where, when, and how he or she receives care. High rates of patient satisfaction and acceptance of VTH have been documented, and studies support the feasibility of using this mode of delivery.[2–4] Also, some patients may feel more comfortable engaging in therapy, or more collaborative within the therapeutic relationship, if a provider is flexible in the ways that he or she is willing to deliver care.[5–9]

Providers delivering care through VTH also may have the advantage of accessing information about the patient's home environment and lifestyle that is not readily available or disclosed during in-person appointments. For example, VTH may better facilitate clinical activities, such as medication reconciliation, assessment of the patient's environment (eg, hoarding), or demonstration of a skill in vivo (eg, practicing exposure exercises). Live access to this type of information also reduces the patient's burden to remember or communicate details of his or her environment relevant to his or her mental health care, allowing more seamless communication between provider and patient. Logistically, VTH saves time for both patient and clinician, by reducing burden of travel and removing administrative aspects of clinical care (eg, checking in during in-person appointments, or picking patients up from the waiting room).

CONSIDERATIONS FOR INCORPORATING VIDEO-TO-HOME TECHNOLOGIES INTO CLINICAL PRACTICE

Despite the many benefits of VTH, some providers express concerns about safety, effectiveness, cost, ease of use, confidentiality, and security. In a recent review of VTH, Fletcher and colleagues[2] explored the literature surrounding the use of VTH for mental health services, with a focus on the following:

- Clinical effectiveness
- Treatment adherence
- Patient and provider satisfaction
- Cost-effectiveness
- Clinical considerations when using VTH
- Implementation of VTH for veterans

Consistent with previous literature,[2] the authors note that VTH is a safe, feasible, and effective option for improving access and maximizing patient choice. Although this body of literature is still growing in response to innovations and improvements in technologies, a consistent message to providers is that they can be confident that delivering care via VTH is comparable and equivalent to in-person care.

With appropriate training and consultation, providers can increase their comfort and competence using VTH. Incorporating VTH into one's practice requires attention to several issues, such as patient appropriateness, setting up the home environment, setting up the required technology, understanding payer models, managing risk remotely, and addressing potential legal and ethical issues. Providers may also have reservations about using technology in their clinical practice for fear of losing control of VTH sessions, concerns about their ability to establish rapport over videoconferencing, and feelings of being ill equipped for safety or emergency situations.[2] Guidance exists on how to address many of these broad issues.[3,10,11] However, the literature does not address additional, more nuanced patient/provider/environmental challenges when using VTH, and they are not always apparent at the outset of treatment. Very few resources discuss relevant clinical considerations for mental health providers wanting to expand their use of VTH beyond basic setup. Thus, many providers may find themselves navigating complex clinical issues throughout treatment, with minimal direction. Of the little work published in this area, much has concentrated on emergency planning and remotely managing patients determined to be high risk for suicidal behaviors, ensuring safety for both patient and provider.[12]

Another limiting factor for some providers may be a lack of understanding about reimbursement models as they relate to VTH services. Insurance coverage and payment issues around telehealth are complex, are rapidly changing, and most often vary by state. Currently, there is no clear guidance on reimbursement for VTH, but around half of all states mandate that reimbursement of telehealth services is comparable to in-person services. Thus, providers should be aware of federal rules and regulations as to what codes may be reimbursed. Although parity exists for telemental health services delivered clinic to clinic, services delivered in-home, such as VTH, are not generally covered; therefore, the extent to which VTH may be reimbursed is unknown. Recommendations include researching policies based on the provider's geographic area and seeking information on insurance company regulations to understand what services and what type of providers are covered and eligible for reimbursement under one's license. That being said, policy changes are happening constantly. For example, effective June 11, 2018, federal legislation known as "Anywhere to Anywhere" was passed, which ". . . ensures that Veterans Affairs healthcare providers can offer the same level of care to all beneficiaries, irrespective of the State or location in a State of the Veterans Affairs health care provider or the beneficiary."[13] Federal support for VTH within the Veterans Health Administration (VHA) waives all copays for VTH sessions. Workload credit for VTH is billed with the same codes and at the same rate as in-person sessions (as long as there is a video component during the session). Although this legislation is not inclusive of providers outside the VHA health care system, it demonstrates the importance of staying aware of the changes in the legal landscape related to VTH.

At present, Medicare, the federal insurance program for those 65 and older and younger people with disabilities, does not cover VTH services. Medicare limits coverage to live video (as opposed to store-and-forward or asynchronous telehealth, or telephone-only services), and the originating site (that is, the location of the patient) must be a rural location, officially designated as a Health Professional Shortage Area or in a county outside a Metropolitan Statistical Area. Moreover, the patient can only be seen in certain medical settings, such as a provider's office, a skilled nursing facility, a rural health clinic, or a hospital.

Because states have more control over their Medicaid programs, nearly all states (49) provide Medicaid coverage for telehealth; around 20% of states provide coverage for store-and-forward services, and nearly half of states do not specify a patient setting or patient location as a condition of payment. Thus, Medicaid is far more flexible than Medicare in reimbursing VTH services right now.

In addition to expanding awareness of the logistics of VTH (eg, getting started, license coverage, insurance reimbursement), clinical fit for this mode of delivery is at the forefront of deciding which patients might benefit most from remotely delivered care. Previously held beliefs about which patient groups are, or are not, a good fit for telehealth are beginning to be challenged.[2] Previous ideas about which patients were inappropriate for telehealth include those with the following:

- Limited access to technology
- Severe psychosis, paranoia, or impaired reality testing
- Poor impulse control or severe mood dysregulation
- Active suicidal or homicidal tendencies
- Active/severe substance use disorder or intoxication
- Severe cognitive impairment
- Severe sensory impairments[3]

With development of new innovations, such as built-in accessibility features for those with sensory impairments, and wider availability of personal technologies (eg, cell phones, tablets) and technologies available through health care systems, many barriers that may have previously limited VTH are no longer an obstacle. These advances, and expansion of the understanding of the safety, effectiveness, and feasibility of VTH, have shifted the field away from an approach of "exclusion criteria," toward an emphasis on clinical expertise of the provider and competency in delivery of VTH.[2]

CLINICAL CHALLENGES AND CREATIVE SOLUTIONS WHEN PROVIDING VIDEO-TO-HOME

This article presents a series of clinical vignettes describing unique challenges providers may face when incorporating VTH into their clinical practice, or when expanding their VTH practice, and offers potential solutions to overcome these barriers. Given that the literature related to VTH is scant, these examples were selected to help providers challenge their biases about what types of patients may be a good fit for VTH. The cases cover 5 issues the authors have encountered when using VTH to deliver mental health care to patients with a wide variety of demographic and clinical characteristics, including the following:

1. Overcoming barriers to technology literacy
2. Increasing access to specialty services for patients living in areas with limited providers
3. Facilitating the transfer of care for patients with complex treatment regimens and logistical barriers to VTH
4. Leveraging VTH to reduce stigma as a barrier to care
5. Remotely managing treatment-interfering behaviors

The authors' primary aim is to increase confidence and competence of providers who are (1) just beginning to use VTH, and (2) looking to expand their clinical offerings to a broader range of patients that includes more challenging clinical populations.

CASE VIGNETTE 1: OVERCOMING BARRIERS TO TECHNOLOGY LITERACY

Continued use of VTH has challenged previously held beliefs and standards regarding which patients are "appropriate" for VTH. Factors, such as age, "tech savviness," and challenging clinical presentations, were previously considered in determinations regarding which patients are best suited for VTH. However, recent studies demonstrate the feasibility of using this approach with a broad selection of patients.[14,15] Moreover, high satisfaction and acceptability of home-based videoconferencing technology are reported across age and other sociodemographic characteristics (eg, rurality[16]). Although additional work toward improving the ease of using technology is needed, the following case vignette demonstrates that level of familiarity with technology and the experience of prior technology problems should not deter providers from offering VTH to patients. Nor should patients be excluded from this type of care, based solely on age, diagnosis, or technological literacy.

A 55-year-old rural veteran with chronic posttraumatic stress disorder (PTSD) characterized by hypervigilance and social isolation was not engaging in VHA clinical services because of a long drive (more than 90 minutes) to the nearest VHA clinic. He also reported experiencing significant anxiety and distress whenever he left his secure home environment. When his provider initially mentioned the option of receiving services directly in his home through VTH, the veteran was hesitant. His previous telehealth experience, limited to clinic-to-clinic videoconferencing, did not leave him with a high level of comfort with navigating technology, nor did it address his travel and anxiety barriers. Despite reservations, the veteran was interested in receiving his care in the comfort of his home through VTH. He was previously dependent on staff assistance to help him navigate telehealth technologies in a clinic setting, but he was willing to try VTH and received a VHA-issued tablet. He had difficulty setting up videoconferencing on the tablet using standard VHA technical support available via phone (National VA Telehealth Helpdesk: 866-651-3180); thus, his provider offered to work with him in person along with the assistance of a remote VHA technical support team to resolve this issue. Although not standard practice, these additional trouble-shooting efforts were time limited and successful. Afterward, the provider created a written technology protocol, specific to the difficulties this patient experienced, that facilitated his use of VTH to engage in ongoing treatment.

CASE VIGNETTE 2: PROVIDING SPECIALIZED MENTAL HEALTH TREATMENT WHEN THERE ARE NO LOCAL PROVIDERS WITH NEEDED EXPERTISE

Given that providers with specialized skill sets tend to be located in larger cities, finding care from a qualified specialty provider may be especially difficult for patients with complex medical and/or psychiatric comorbidities who live in rural areas.[17] The following case vignette showcases how VTH can be used to increase access to specialty mental health services for rural and underserved patients.

A 17-year-old female student from a rural area was hospitalized following her first manic episode while at college. Upon her discharge from the hospital, her family was unable to find local providers who could provide follow-up care, particularly for an adolescent suffering from bipolar disorder. As a result, the family had to drive 3 hours to the university clinic, where the patient received medication management and the family engaged in specialty psychotherapy for bipolar disorder from experts in child and adolescent bipolar disorder. Concerned about the sustainability of traveling nearly 6 hours round trip for future appointments, the patient, family, and providers discussed the option of receiving care via telehealth. Via VTH, the patient continued to see her psychiatrist every few months for ongoing medication management, and the family continued in family therapy, psychoeducation, and relapse prevention training for bipolar disorder. When family therapy was completed, the adolescent was able to continue seeing her therapist via VTH for individual therapy.

CASE VIGNETTE 3: NAVIGATING CONTINUITY OF CARE UPON LOSING A PROVIDER

As shown above, VTH can reduce many logistical barriers to receiving care (eg, distance to provider, work schedule) and provide access to specialty care that otherwise may not be available within a geographic area. Even in routine clinical practice, patients can have complex treatment regimens that require specialized training or clinical experience. This can make transferring these patients' care to another provider very challenging following the loss of a primary provider. The following case vignette shows why VTH may be a valuable solution in this scenario.

A 64-year-old woman living in a rural community had been receiving in-person care for 20+ years from a psychiatrist 1 hour away, for long-standing depression. Although she was only seen every 3 to 4 months, the patient was on a medication regimen that included a monoamine oxidase inhibitor and an antipsychotic, as well as medications for diabetes and hypertension. After numerous failed trials on selective serotonin reuptake inhibitors, selective norepinephrine reuptake inhibitors, and tricyclic antidepressants, the patient began taking tranylcypromine, which, combined with olanzapine, led to complete remission of her depressive symptoms. When it was almost time for her provider to retire, they discussed the patient's need for another provider who was both knowledgeable and comfortable with complex medication regimens such as hers.

During their discussion, the patient was adamant about not wanting to change medications, fearing a relapse of her depression. In agreement, her psychiatrist contacted her primary care provider about transferring her care. Her primary care provider was willing to bridge the patient's medications for a few months but felt uncomfortable prescribing and monitoring a complex psychiatric medication regimen that included a monoamine oxidase inhibitor. At their next appointment, the psychiatrist and patient discussed seeing a specialist in mood disorders at a nearby university. Her psychiatrist was aware that the patient's husband's health had steadily deteriorated to the point where she was unable leave him alone for the full day it would take her to drive to the nearest major city, see a psychiatrist, and return home. Luckily, the mood disorder specialist at the university was willing to see the patient via VTH. The patient was thankful that she would be able to continue her medication regimen while staying home to care for her husband.

CASE VIGNETTE 4: LEVERAGING VIDEO-TO-HOME TO OVERCOME STIGMA

Self-imposed and social stigmas about mental health are major barriers to care.[18] Mental health stigma perpetuates negative stereotypes that diminish help seeking, especially in public domains. VTH technology places practitioners in a unique position to deliver health care to stigmatized populations that might not otherwise receive treatment. VTH also provides a sense of security for patients because they can control the environment in which treatment is received. The following case vignette illustrates the use of VTH to promote treatment engagement among patients who might not otherwise engage in care because of stigma-related barriers.

A 28-year-old female veteran was referred for treatment to address chronic PTSD symptoms associated with military sexual trauma. During intake, she appeared visibly anxious. When her therapist asked about her demeanor, the veteran shared that coming to the VHA was difficult. She often felt that people knew she had been assaulted and were silently judging her. She was also uncomfortable sitting in clinic waiting rooms, predominantly occupied by male veterans. This heightened her fears of potentially confronting her perpetrator or even being assaulted again. Sensitive to these concerns, the veteran and her therapist opted for VTH delivery of Prolonged Exposure, a well-established PTSD treatment that has been successfully delivered through VTH technology.[19–21]

The veteran initially received VTH sessions in her apartment, where she resided alone. Concerned that her neighbors could overhear her sessions, she wore headphones and occasionally used the built-in chat-room feature to discuss very private information. This feature was most helpful when assessing her symptoms at each session. Part of the veteran's treatment included in vivo exposure, during which the therapist helps the patient approach anxiety-provoking situations without performing avoidance strategies that would otherwise further reinforce anxiety. In preparation for the behavioral exposures, the veteran's therapist saw an opportunity to provide her with real-time feedback that could optimize her therapeutic experience. At the next session, the veteran checked in with her therapist from her parked car to review the exposure, which involved walking in a crowded park. Afterward, the veteran reconnected with her therapist from the car to debrief and receive feedback. She completed the remaining in vivo exposures on her own, between therapy sessions. As she grew confident with using her newly acquired skills in her daily life, she and her therapist moved toward a hybrid approach in which the veteran attended a mixture of in-person and VTH sessions. This promoted generalization of her skills to different environments and situations. At their terminating session, the veteran thanked her therapist for recommending VTH, admitting that she would have dropped out of treatment if in-person sessions were her only option. She noted that the virtual space created a physical buffer that made it easier to engage with the provider without ruminating on the therapist's perceptions of her.

CASE VIGNETTE 5: REMOTELY MANAGING TREATMENT-INTERFERING BEHAVIORS

Behaviors disruptive to the therapeutic relationship, otherwise known as treatment-interfering behaviors, range in intent or purpose, may be overt or covert, and can be directed toward the self or others.[22] Common examples include homework noncompliance, missing sessions, frequently switching the focus of therapy, or withholding information or disclosing nonfactual information. These behaviors are often defined by their function rather than intent and make it difficult for the patient to effectively and successfully engage in treatment. For example, missed sessions may reflect avoidance behavior or possible disagreement with the treatment approach. Although the aforementioned behaviors may present during VTH delivery, nonverbal behavior is often less pronounced or more ambiguous when using VTH technology. This can make it difficult to recognize when a disruptive behavior is occurring. There may also be technology-specific disruptive behaviors to manage that are not applicable to in-person settings (eg, intermittently and/or unexpectedly turning off the camera or audio, scheduling appointments at inappropriate times). New, creative solutions for addressing these therapy-interfering behaviors over VTH, as presented in the following case vignette, may be needed.

A 46-year-old man was receiving individual psychotherapy to address his history of complex trauma beginning in childhood. Early in treatment, he canceled or missed in-person appointments frequently owing to last-minute shift changes at work. He worked a variable schedule at a part-time job, filling in shifts whenever he could to make a livable wage. He and his provider discussed using VTH, which was expected to accommodate his variable work schedule. Agreeable with this plan, the patient was easily able to set up his personal iPad to connect with his provider. However, during the second session, he ended the encounter early to take a work-related call. With the progression of sessions, more and more interruptions disturbed scheduled sessions. For example, the patient once connected to a session while operating equipment in the warehouse and another time while driving on the highway. This behavioral pattern concerned the provider, especially because these behaviors escalated. Not only was the patient putting himself in a vulnerable and unsafe position (eg, answering while driving and operating heavy machinery), but he was also violating the provider's boundaries in a way that could have legal implications (eg, malpractice lawsuit). At the next session, the patient answered the phone while putting on his work shirt. The provider spent that session identifying the patient's therapy-interfering behaviors, also exploring prompting events; consequences of the behavior; and alternative, more skillful behaviors. One solution they generated included moving sessions from unstructured home and work environments to a predetermined private space in a public setting easily accessible to him. Rather than delaying the start of time of visits, the provider encouraged the patient to use skillful strategies, such as verbalizing discomfort, which complemented the mode of delivery because there were fewer opportunities to interpret nonverbal behaviors. The therapist reasserted therapy boundaries by collaboratively generating a contract of "ground rules" for the way sessions would continue (eg, not connecting while driving), with consequences that the sessions would be rescheduled rather than delayed. Finding stability in location and clarity in therapeutic boundaries allowed greater structure of therapy sessions, while still offering a flexible approach to the patient.

CLINICAL LESSONS LEARNED FROM VIRTUAL HOUSE CALLS IN MENTAL HEALTH

In the first case vignette, it was learned that generating guidelines for patients without strong technical skills may help patients overcome barriers related to technology literacy. Patients who appear to be poor candidates for in-home videoconferencing because of a lack of technological acumen may be able to participate with additional setup support and training from providers. Operating from the position that patients can learn to navigate new technologies will help challenge providers' misconceptions about the need for patients to be "tech savvy." Relatedly, the way a provider explains or describes VTH to patients, otherwise known as "messaging," will influence patients' confidence and willingness to engage in this mode of delivery. Providers may benefit from exploring their messaging of VTH to patients and take note of discrepancies in explaining the VTH approach, which may lead to disparities in whom is offered this type of care (eg, older adults). Providers who engage their patients in a collaborative process of troubleshooting around technology may also find this process helps establish, build, and strengthen rapport. These suggestions should be considered in the context of both time and effort available from the organization (eg, resources to develop training materials) to provide this type of support as well as the overall potential benefit to the patient.

The second and third vignettes offer snapshots of how VTH can eliminate barriers to engaging in traditional mental health services. These cases, although seemingly at opposite ends of the spectrum (eg, engaging an adolescent in family-centered care vs assisting an older adult in replacing access to specialty mental health), have many overlapping themes. VTH reduces the overall burden of care for patients living in areas with limited access to specialty care for serious mental illness (eg, bipolar disorder) or chronic psychiatric disorders. It can improve integrated health care services whenever patients can see members of their treatment team, increasing the sustainability of complex treatment regimens (eg, psychiatry visits, family therapy sessions, individual sessions). Allowing patients to be seen in their homes also addresses many practical barriers (eg, traveling long distances to nearest facility, caregiving responsibilities), which increases engagement and fosters support.

In the fourth case vignette, adapting the patient's treatment environment helped to overcome stigma and enhance exposure-based work, leading to better outcomes. This flexible approach gives stigmatized patients a sense of control over their environment. The virtual space can reduce concerns about public ridicule and privacy and create an environment in which the patient is better able to engage in treatment. Furthermore, this case demonstrated how VTH can enhance elements of a treatment protocol that are not easily replicated in the traditional office-based therapeutic environment (eg, conducting live exposures in the patients' natural environments). In other words, providers are not restricted to the patients' home or office setting.

The final case vignette provided insight into how providers might address treatment-interfering behaviors over VTH. VTH introduces new ways for sessions to be disrupted and, therefore, providers must expand their understanding of what constitutes a treatment-interfering behavior (eg, poor eye contact vs deliberately positioning oneself off camera). These behaviors may also be difficult to detect, because VTH affords less access to nonverbal communication. Therapists should use a collaborative therapeutic process to identify these behaviors with the patient and integrate the solution into ongoing therapy when possible. Therapeutic techniques used during in-person encounters can help inform and model a virtual approach, such as structuring contingencies.

All in all, providers may need to get creative when incorporating VTH into their clinical practice. Evidence-based guidelines, tools, and techniques commonly recommended for in-person encounters can likely be adapted to VTH. That being said, VTH should be conceptualized as the mode in which a provider is delivering a treatment rather than the treatment itself. It may also be helpful to think about VTH as a clinical tool that can be combined with more traditional in-person models of care. This point of view allows a provider the flexibility to offer "hybrid-style" care, whereby a provider may use VTH to bridge between less frequent in-person sessions, or as a way to enhance treatment protocols (eg, exposure-based therapies).

SUMMARY

As the understanding of clinical appropriateness for VTH expands, so does the capacity of providers to deliver patient-centered care that can be tailored to the specific needs of individual patients. VTH also allows greater flexibility in how, when, and where services are received, which may add to the collaborative nature of the therapeutic process. Connecting to patients electronically, in their homes, affords greater access to information about patients' environments that otherwise might not be disclosed and can enhance the quality of care by increasing generalizability of skills to different contexts.

Technology is allowing providers to expand their reach and deepen clinical experiences through the use of enhanced features. For example, clinical conditions once deemed inappropriate for VTH (eg, substance use disorders, psychosis, sensory impairments) are no longer exclusionary criteria for providers with expertise in those areas who wish to reach their patient via VTH.[2] Enhanced built-in features of VTH, such as chat rooms, offer greater opportunity for self-disclosure for patients with privacy concerns. More importantly, the option to incorporate standard accessibility features, such as Bluetooth technology or screen-reading features, is useful to patients with sensory impairments and physical limitations. It is important for providers to remain aware of these available features and make them accessible to patients to facilitate provision of care via VTH.

The authors are hopeful that their case vignettes will challenge thoughts about who may be a good fit for VTH and expand providers' consideration of this mode of delivery for a broader array of patients. Their goal is to increase comfort and competence of VTH among both new and well-practiced providers. There are additional resources that may provide further study on case vignettes and to also help providers get "up and running" (please see Campbell, and colleagues[10] and American Telemedicine Association[23]). Continued education and training will facilitate greater comfort and competence with this mode of delivery. The authors recommend generating or joining a community of practice of other VTH providers, which will continue to foster increased comfort and confidence with VTH as well as help facilitate the exchange of information among new and established providers.

REFERENCES

1. Lindsay JA, Hudson S, Martin L, et al. Implementing video to home to increase access to evidence-based psychotherapy for rural veterans. J Technol Behav Sci 2017;2(3–4):140–8.
2. Fletcher TL, Hogan J, Keegan F, et al. Recent advances in delivering mental health treatment via video to home. Curr Psychiatry Rep 2018;20:56.
3. Morland LA, Poizer JM, Williams KE, et al. Home-based clinical video teleconferencing care: clinical consideration and future directions. Int Rev Psychiatry 2015; 27(6):504–12.
4. Shore P, Goranson A, Ward MF, et al. Meeting Veterans where they're @: a VA home-based telemental health (HBTMH) pilot program. Int J Psychiatry Med 2014;48(1):5–17.

5. Paris MB, Fazio S, Chan S, et al. Managing psychiatrist-patient relationship in the digital age: a summary review of the impact of technology-enabled care on clinical processes and rapport. Curr Psychiatry Rep 2017;19:90.

6. Murdoch JW, Connor-Greene PA. Enhancing therapeutic impact and therapeutic alliance through electronic mail homework assignments. J Psychother Pract Res 2000;9:232–7.

7. Sucala M, Schnur J, Constantino MJ, et al. The therapeutic relationship in e-therapy for mental health: a systematic review. J Med Internet Res 2012;14(4): e110, p.2.

8. Lozano BE, Birks AH, Kloezeman K, et al. Therapeutic alliance in clinical videoconferencing; optimizing the communication context. In: Tuerk P, Shore P, editors. Clinical videoconferencing in telehealth: program developments and practice. New York: Springer Publications; 2014. p. 221–51.

9. Goldstein F, Glueck D. Developing rapport and therapeutic alliance during telemental health sessions with children and adolescents. J Child Adolesc Psychopharmacol 2016;26(3):204–11.

10. Campbell LF, Millán F, Martin JN, editors. A telepsychology casebook: using technology ethically and effectively in your professional practice. Washington, DC: American Psychological Association; 2018.

11. Yellowlees P, Shore JH. Telepsychiatry and health technologies: a guide for mental health professionals. Washington, DC: American Psychiatric Publications; 2018.

12. Shore P, Lu M. Patient safety planning and emergency management. In: Tuerk P, Shore P, editors. Clinical videoconferencing in telehealth: program developments and practice. New York: Springer Publications; 2014. p. 167–201.

13. Department of Veterans Affairs. Federal Register 2018;83(92) Friday, May 11, 2018. Rules and regulations. 38 CFR Part 17, RIN 2900-AQ06, "Authority of Health Care Providers to Practice Telehealth."

14. Choi NG, Marti CN, Bruce ML, et al. Six-month post-intervention depression and disability outcomes of in-home telehealth problem-solving therapy for depressed, low-income homebound older adults. Depress Anxiety 2014;31(8):653–61.

15. King VL, Brooner RK, Peirce JM, et al. A randomized trial of web-based videoconferencing for substance abuse counseling. J Subst Abuse Treat 2014;46:36–42.

16. Richardson LK, Frueh CB, Grubaugh AL, et al. Current directions in videoconferencing tele-mental health research. Clin Psychol (New York) 2010;16(3):323–38.

17. Durland L, Interian A, Pretzer-Aboff I, et al. Effect of telehealth-to-home interventions on quality of life for individuals with depressive and anxiety disorders. Ment Health Care 2014;9:12.

18. Corrigan PW, Druss BG, Perlick DA. The impact of mental illness stigma on seeking and participating in mental health care. Psychol Sci Public Interest 2014;15(2):37–70.

19. Gros DF, Lancaster CL, Lopez CM, et al. Treatment satisfaction of home-based telehealth exposure for combat-related PTSD in veterans. J Telemed Telecare 2018;24(1):51–5.

20. Acierno R, Knapp R, Tuerk P, et al. A non-inferiority trial of prolonged exposure for posttraumatic stress disorder: in person versus home-based telehealth. Behav Res Ther 2017;89:57–65.

21. Yuen EK, Gros DF, Price M, et al. Randomized controlled trial of home-based telehealth versus in-person prolonged exposure for combat-related PTSD in Veterans: preliminary results. J Clin Psychol 2015;71(6):500–12.

22. Linehan MM. Cognitive behavioral treatment of borderline personality disorder. New York: Guildford Publications; 2018.
23. American Telemedicine Association practice guidelines for video-based online mental health services. 2013. Available at: http://www.armericantelemed.org. resources/standards/ata-standards-guidelines/practice-guidelines-for-video-bas ed-online-mental-health-services. Accessed February 26, 2019.

Recommendations for Using Clinical Video Telehealth with Patients at High Risk for Suicide

Meghan M. McGinn, PhD[a,b],*, Milena S. Roussev, PhD[a],
Erika M. Shearer, PhD[c], Russell A. McCann, PhD[b,c],
Sasha M. Rojas, MS[a,d], Bradford L. Felker, MD[a,b]

KEYWORDS

- Telemedicine • Suicide • Mental health services • Access to health care

KEY POINTS

- Clinical video telehealth (CVT) has the potential to deliver much-needed mental health services to individuals at risk for suicide who face access barriers.
- None of the literature, professional guidelines, and laws pertaining to the provision of mental health services via CVT suggest that high-risk patients should be excluded from this modality.
- Best practices for assessment and management of suicide risk can be feasibly performed by mental health professionals via CVT.
- Mental health professionals delivering services via CVT to high-risk patients would benefit from a multidisciplinary network of CVT providers for referral and consultation.

There is a growing body of evidence supporting the safe and effective use of clinical video telehealth (CVT) in the provision of mental health services,[1,2] and the benefits of using this modality, including increasing access and reducing rates of hospitalization,

Disclosure: The authors have no relationships with any commercial company that has a direct financial interest in the subject matter or materials discussed in this article or with a company making a competing product. The views expressed in this article are those of the authors and do not necessarily reflect the position or policy of the Department of Veterans Affairs or the United States government.
[a] VA Puget Sound Health Care System, S-116-MHC, 1660 South Columbian Way, Seattle, WA 98108, USA; [b] Department of Psychiatry and Behavioral Sciences, University of Washington School of Medicine, 1959 NE Pacific St, Seattle, WA, USA; [c] VA Puget Sound Health Care System, A-116-VIP, 9600 Veterans Drive Southwest, Tacoma, WA 98493, USA; [d] University of Arkansas, Fayetteville, AR, USA
* Corresponding author. VA Puget Sound Health Care System, S-116-MHC, 1660 South Columbian Way, Seattle, WA 98108.
E-mail address: meghan.mcginn@va.gov

Psychiatr Clin N Am 42 (2019) 587–595
https://doi.org/10.1016/j.psc.2019.08.009
0193-953X/19/© 2019 Elsevier Inc. All rights reserved.

have been widely cited.[3–5] At the same time, there remains concern among many providers about the use of CVT, particularly for those patients considered at high risk for suicide.[6] This concern creates a juxtaposition such that the patients who are most in need of access to mental health services are often excluded from using CVT because of provider perceptions that the modality is not appropriate for high risk patients.

The current article (1) reviews the body of published studies, professional guidelines, and laws that pertain to the use of CVT with patients at high risk for suicide, and (2) provides practical recommendations for how to adapt best-practice guidelines for assessing and managing suicide risk when treating high-risk patients for the CVT modality. The authors are providers with extensive experience in the provision of mental health treatment via CVT within the Veterans Administration (VA) health care system, and case examples are included to show the recommended adaptations for using this modality in the assessment and management of individuals at high risk for suicide.

RESEARCH EVIDENCE FOR THE USE OF CLINICAL VIDEO TELEHEALTH WITH HIGH-RISK PATIENTS

There is strong evidence to suggest the equivalency of mental health services delivered via CVT compared with in-person delivery; however, many clinical trials have excluded participants who were considered high risk.[1,2,7] There is not 1 randomized control trial (RCT) that examines the effects of CVT, compared with in-person treatment, on clinical risk outcomes among high-risk populations. Secondary analysis from a recent RCT suggests individuals who presented with greater levels of hopelessness at baseline were likely to improve more if they completed in-person treatment compared with CVT, although both groups did improve after treatment.[8] It is clear that the field would benefit from research that is more inclusive of high-risk individuals and that directly studies risk outcomes.

At the same time, the literature to date does provide evidence that emergency situations that arise in the context of therapy can be successfully managed via CVT,[9] and CVT has been effectively used in the assessment and treatment of psychiatric emergency patients[10] as well as persons in rural shelters after experiencing domestic violence.[11] Furthermore, in a study examining clinical outcomes of patients enrolled in CVT services between 2006 and 2010, Godleski and colleagues[3] found a 25% decrease in hospitalizations among veterans receiving care via CVT, and, among those who were admitted, they observed a decrease in days of psychiatric hospitalization. There is also evidence outside the VA system that CVT can help reduce rehospitalization within a 12-month period and increase treatment adherence in rural patients following psychiatric hospitalization.[12] In summary, although there is a lack of clinical trial data that specifically target high-risk patients, there are observable benefits of this modality and a precedent for how to manage risk safely.

Some investigators have speculated that CVT offers some unique benefits for suicide assessment compared with care as usual, which is often telephone-based risk assessment. For example, Godleski and colleagues[13] note that CVT (1) offers visual cues about the patients' emotional states, (2) allows for suicide assessments in remote areas where providers may not be available, (3) can reduce the need for hospitalization when effective treatments can be provided via CVT, and (4) can allow culturally sensitive care to be delivered, particularly where language barriers might be present. Pruitt and collegues[5] reviewed clinical benefits of CVT to the home, in which veterans received mental health services directly into their homes. They argue that CVT may enhance safety for both patients and practitioners, such that collaboratively establishing a safety plan with the patient may in itself offer therapeutic benefits.

PROFESSIONAL GUIDELINES REGARDING THE USE OF CLINICAL VIDEO TELEHEALTH

Practice standards and guidelines relevant to providing CVT services to high-risk patients have been published by various professional associations, including the National Association of Social Workers[14] and American Psychological Association (APA),[15] as well as a joint taskforce comprising the American Psychiatric Association and American Telemedicine Association (ATA).[16] None of these guidelines identify a circumstance in which using the CVT modality in practice would always be contraindicated. Instead, these guidelines focus on offering various considerations that may affect the determination of whether CVT would be clinically appropriate for patients.

Identified factors to consider when determining the appropriateness include patients' cognitive capacity, history of cooperation, history of substance use, history of violence or self-injurious behavior, and nearby community resources (eg, hospitals, clinics, laboratories). In addition, patients should understand that CVT could be discontinued at any time, and that they may need to present in person to a clinic as part of the services offered (eg, physical examination, laboratory services). Collectively, these considerations are less salient when patients are seen via CVT while seated in a supervised setting (eg, at a rural clinic with medical support staff). Such sites may have ample medical resources that clinicians can leverage to support their patients. The aforementioned considerations for determining appropriateness of patients may carry more importance when patients are seen in nonclinic locations, such as their homes, vehicles, places of work, or other unsupervised locales. When clinical resources are not available during the encounter to conduct physical examinations and laboratory tests, and staff are not nearby to assist with emergency interventions, the importance of patient cooperativeness, such as their willingness to engage in suitable clinical alternatives and follow safety plans, becomes paramount.

These professional associations' guidelines separately address discipline-specific topics that are relevant to working with high-risk patients. For example, the 2018 APA/ATA guidelines speak to the prescription of controlled substances via CVT[16] and the 2013 APA guidelines discuss the use of test and assessment instruments over this modality.[15] However, there are also common themes across guidelines, such as the importance of a patient-specific emergency plan and the acknowledgment that patients' appropriateness for CVT may change over time.[14–16]

LAWS AFFECTING PROVISION OF CLINICAL VIDEO TELEHEALTH TO HIGH-RISK INDIVIDUALS

On a federal level, the Ryan Haight Act[17] affects psychiatric care for all patients by restricting the prescribing of controlled substances via CVT in certain contexts. A detailed overview of the Ryan Haight Act is beyond the scope of this article, and although there are additional exceptions, the Ryan Haight Act generally requires that providers prescribing a controlled substance via CVT either must have previously seen their patients once in person or their patients must be physically located at a Drug Enforcement Administration (DEA)–registered facility at the time of the prescription event. The Ryan Haight Act is not specific to care for high-risk patients; however, it does make it so psychiatric providers may be unable to prescribe in the same way via CVT as they might in person, creating a situation in which caring for high-risk patients via CVT could be affected such that it would be preferable to meet in person, or at least via another, legally tenable CVT arrangement that allows patients to receive the appropriate level of care (eg, while the patient is located at a DEA-registered clinic). It seems that the Ryan Haight Act's impact on CVT will soon change. In October 2018, the

Substance Use–Disorder Prevention that Promotes Opioid Recovery and Treatment (SUPPORT) for Patients and Communities Act[18] was signed into law, which will require the United States Attorney General to implement a process for providers to register as exempt from restrictions put forth by the Ryan Haight Act, effectively enabling them to practice via CVT in a manner more consistent with in-person care. The Attorney General has until October 2019 to put this registration process into effect. The authors think that implementation of the SUPPORT Act will better enable providers to work with more varied clinical presentations via CVT, including those with higher risk.

State law also affects working with high-risk patients via CVT. Each state has laws that regulate the provision of CVT to patients physically located in the respective state. In general, providers need to be licensed in each state they support via CVT. Some states require that providers seek full licenses to practice via CVT, whereas some states offer CVT-specific licenses, and still other states have various mechanisms designed to both encourage and regulate providers from out of state serving patients in their area. Under a recent amendment to its medical regulations,[19] the VA health care system has ruled that providers are able to engage in interstate CVT practice without being licensed in more than 1 location; however, regardless, all providers may still be held liable to the laws of the state where their patients are seated. Providers may also be held liable to states where they are physically located as well.[13] Practically speaking, if providers are only licensed in 1 state and provide CVT within that same state, they need only to become familiar with that state's laws related to both mental health care broadly and CVT. If providers are licensed and practicing via CVT in multiple states, they need to be fully aware of the legal differences that exist between states, and adjust their practices accordingly. For example, providers might follow a certain process for getting patients involuntarily committed in one state, and be required to follow still a different commitment process in another state. If laws for providers' locations are not congruent, providers might be wise to proceed cautiously. The implications of varied state law have a major impact on working with high-risk patients.

ADAPTING BEST-PRACTICE GUIDELINES FOR WORKING WITH HIGH-RISK PATIENTS TO CLINICAL VIDEO TELEHEALTH DELIVERY

The literature, professional guidelines, and laws discussed earlier may heavily inform the provision of CVT to high-risk patients, but none of them suggest that CVT services should not be offered for such clinical presentations. As such, the second aim of this article is to discuss how to adapt best-practice guidelines for working with high-risk patients to CVT delivery of these services. Through a collaborative effort, the Department of Defense (DOD) and the VA developed the Clinical Practice Guideline for the Assessment and Management of Suicide Risk.[20] This guideline provides evidence-based recommendations and a structured framework for assessing suicide risk and facilitating hospitalization when warranted. The VA/DOD defines high-acute risk for suicide as individuals with persistent suicidal ideation, strong suicidal intention or plan, poor impulse control, or a recent suicide attempt or preparatory behavior, and identifies hospitalization as the first-line recommended treatment of such high-acute–risk individuals. Although there is not a CVT application analogous to inpatient care, providers may encounter patients at high risk for suicide via CVT during the assessment phase or after discharge. A discussion of how to adapt the VA/DOD recommendations to the CVT modality when working with high-risk patients is presented later (in bulleted points), accompanied by case examples from the authors' clinical experiences and informed by the extant literature and the professional guidelines mentioned earlier for use of CVT.

Assessment

The recommendations in the VA/DOD's Clinical Practice Guideline for the Assessment and Management of Suicide Risk[20] include the completion of a comprehensive assessment of suicide risk by a behavioral health provider. As in the case of in-person treatment, suicide risk assessment via the CVT modality may include data from several sources; for example, routinely administered screening measures as a part of measurement-based care (eg, Patient Health Questionnaire); visual cues that may indicate depressed mood; collateral reports from loved ones; and the patients' own verbal reports.

Although many elements of the assessment will be the same via CVT as in person, consider the following adaptations:

- To ensure patient safety, obtain the patients' location at the start of the interaction to allow for enacting an emergency plan.
- Consider HIPAA (Health Insurance Portability and Accountability Act)-compliant options for sending and receiving written questionnaires (eg, secure messaging, postal mail, patient holding completed measure up to the screen).
- If the patient is located out of state, familiarize yourself with the laws of that state, such as for involuntary commitment and abuse reporting.

Hospitalization

When a comprehensive risk assessment via CVT reveals that hospitalization is indicated, there are a few CVT-related considerations for facilitating this process:

- Remain connected with the patient via CVT throughout the process of coordinating hospitalization. If the connection is lost, try to reconnect via CVT or call the patient on the phone.
- While maintaining the CVT call, either the provider or the patient can call emergency services by telephone to coordinate involvement of emergency services for transport, if necessary.
- Use the support of other staff to assist with patient care coordination during the CVT call (eg, use the phone, pager, or internal instant messaging system to connect with suicide prevention coordinators, colleagues, or other support staff). Secondary support staff may be able to assist with contacting emergency departments or emergency services, or simply provide consultation in real time allowing the provider to document peer concurrence with the steps taken to ensure patient safety.
- Work with other individuals present in the home as needed.

Case Example: Assessment and Hospitalization via Clinical Video Telehealth

During a home-based CVT appointment, a 33-year-old divorced male veteran stated that he "just can't take it anymore" and discussed his concerns related to suicide. Through assessment, it was deemed that the veteran was at imminent risk for suicide and that his risk level warranted a higher level of care. The veteran was amenable to hospitalization. Because the veteran was at home, did not have a support person nearby to drive him to the hospital, and was not able to drive himself, the decision was made to contact emergency services for immediate evaluation and transport to the local hospital emergency department. The veteran was given the option of either calling the 911 himself or having his provider call 911, both while maintaining CVT connection with this provider. The veteran opted to call 911 himself. He maintained the CVT connection while he called 911 so that this provider could continue to observe and hear the interaction. While waiting for emergency services to arrive, the veteran continued with his provider and was able to engage in grounding techniques and discuss coordination of care related to the hospitalization.

When emergency services arrived, the veteran was able to introduce his provider to emergency services personnel via CVT, and together they discussed the clinical situation. The veteran was voluntarily hospitalized because of acute suicidal risk.

Determining the Appropriate Setting and Modality of Care After Discharge

The VA/DOD clinical practice guideline states that once an individual no longer has suicidal intent, has obtained a level of psychiatric stability (eg, is no longer intoxicated or acutely psychotic), and is willing and able to perform a safety plan, the patient should be moved to a less restrictive setting of care.[20] For individuals with access barriers, CVT is an appealing option as a less restrictive setting for outpatient care. However, because CVT is only a modality of care and not a specific treatment in itself, consider the following:

- First, consider what level of care and type of treatment is clinically indicated for the patient. For example, if substance use is a strong risk factor, consider referral to a substance use disorders program, or, if borderline personality disorder is the underlying disorder contributing to risk, consider referral to a full dialectical behavioral therapy (DBT[21]) program.
- Once referred to the appropriate clinical setting, then consider the appropriateness for delivering treatment via CVT in this setting. At a minimum, the patients need to be willing to follow through on a CVT-specific safety plan, meaning they must be willing to provide a location at each session so that the provider may activate the emergency plan as needed. The safety plan may also include limiting access to means during sessions to ensure that it is a safe setting for treatment.
- Note that not every high-risk patient is appropriate for CVT. Providers are encouraged to consider each high-risk patient on a case-by-case basis, and consult with colleagues when making this determination.

Case Example: Determining Appropriateness for Outpatient Treatment via Clinical Video Telehealth

A rurally located, 80-year-old veteran was referred for anger management. The veteran requested CVT to home, because he reportedly never leaves his house because of fear that he will end up hurting someone. He described to the referring provider, a primary care mental health provider at the community-based outpatient clinic, that he carries a loaded weapon with him at all times and that once in the past month he pointed the weapon at his own head when experiencing high distress. He did not have active suicidal ideation, plan, or intent at the time of referral, but he described having low frustration tolerance, and acknowledged that technology failure is a trigger for distress. The veteran also expressed that he did not want to work on learning skills that will help him to manage his anger and be able to leave his home, but rather wanted therapy that would allow him to "vent." Because of his belief that it keeps him safer to carry a weapon, he was unwilling to restrict access to his weapon during sessions. The details of this referral were discussed with the CVT team. Because technology failure, a trigger for the veteran's distress, is a common occurrence during CVT sessions and the veteran described a history of impulsive suicidal behavior (eg, holding a gun to his head) in the context of distress, it was determined that the CVT modality may put him at greater risk. The team recommended that the referring provider consider referral to a residential program or other in-person treatment, or, if the patient is truly unwilling to leave the house, consider whether telephone may be a more appropriate modality because it is less prone to technology failure.

Ongoing Management of Patients at Risk for Suicide in an Outpatient Setting

The VA/DOD clinical practice guideline for managing patients at risk for suicide suggests that the first goal of treatment with high-risk patients should be to secure patient safety by addressing the following: patient and family education, limiting access to lethal means, safety planning, addressing psychosocial risk factors, and documenting a rationale and treatment plan.[20] As is the case for assessment, most patient management via the CVT modality is congruent with the in-person modality, but the following adaptations should be considered:

- Suggest inviting family members to a video visit with the patient to provide family education. If they are already present in the home, this may be more easily accomplished via CVT.
- Include creating a safe space for treatment in discussion of access to lethal means. Use the ability for patients to show you their environment to help set up a safe space.
- A copy of the safety plan can be mailed/sent via secure messaging or a blank safety plan provided ahead of time for the patient to fill out.
- Include in informed consent that CVT may be discontinued if it is determined to be an unsafe or ineffective modality for the patient.

Other best-practice recommendations for managing high-risk patients include addressing psychosocial risk factors, offering evidence-based therapies that target suicide risk, considering pharmacotherapies that have been shown to reduce suicide risk in the case of specific underlying disorders, and increasing engagement with strategies such as case care management.[20] These recommendations are most efficiently performed with a team approach to treatment of high-risk patients, providing these patients with access to multiple disciplines (social workers, psychiatrists, psychologists, nurse care-managers) and providers with different areas of expertise. As such, the authors recommend:

- In large systems of care, train full interdisciplinary teams in the use of telehealth technologies in order to provide patient access to multiple resources and team support for the providers managing risk remotely.
- For providers operating independently, it is prudent to network with others who provide telemental health to ensure the availability of case consultation with peers who also have experience using the modality and the ability to refer to appropriate treatment if the patient's treatment needs change.
- If medications are indicated, consider implication of Ryan Haight Act[17] and eventually the SUPPORT Act.[18]
- Consider augmenting or following up treatment via CVT with telephone care management or electronic symptom monitoring.

Case Example: Ongoing Management of Risk via Clinical Video Telehealth Following Inpatient Discharge

A 47-year-old partnered male veteran was discharged from a 72-hour hospitalization following a recent suicide attempt. He was discharged back to his home-based CVT provider with whom he been engaged in biweekly treatment of posttraumatic stress disorder (PTSD). The veteran was unsure regarding whether he had suicidal intent because he had been so intoxicated that he could not remember whether his intention was to commit suicide or to serve as a cry for help. The veteran's distance from the VA as well as his lack of driver's license because of a previous conviction for driving under the influence made access to in-person treatment difficult. His substance use and abuse were assessed and it was determined that his alcohol use had increased dramatically and warranted additional treatment beyond his current provider's expertise. The veteran's home-based CVT provider consulted with the local VA addictions treatment center (ATC) regarding coordinating care. A plan was made for the veteran to meet with a provider on the ATC team for home-based treatment via CVT in addition to his PTSD treatment to increase the level of care because of his recent hospitalization as well as to provide alcohol use disorder treatment. The ATC provider was able to coordinate with a community-based outpatient clinic to collect urinalysis as necessary. Ultimately, after some work with the veteran, he was amenable to engaging in residential treatment of alcohol use disorder and PTSD. On discharge from the residential programs, he resumed home-based treatment with both his ATC and PTSD providers via CVT.

SUMMARY AND FUTURE DIRECTIONS

The present article summarizes the literature, professional guidelines, and laws pertaining to the delivery of mental health services to patients at high risk for suicide. Although more research is still needed, these sources are generally supportive of caring for high-risk patients via CVT. Many of the existing clinical practice guidelines for assessing and managing suicide risk can feasibly be performed with minor modification.

Future research should specifically address the effectiveness of interventions delivered via CVT at reducing suicide risk factors. Likewise, to our knowledge, CVT delivery of several of the recommended treatment options for suicide risk and underlying disorders (eg, DBT for borderline personality disorder[21]) have not yet been implemented and evaluated. However, existing research does provide evidence that providers can effectively manage acute emergencies remotely and that many patients benefit from treatments delivered via CVT.

Provider concerns about CVT with high-risk patients are still prevalent,[6] and thus it is important to consider how to support providers in managing risk remotely. The VA health care system, because of the larger quantity of trained providers, can provide some models for this type of support that could be applied to non-VA settings. For example, every VA medical center hires suicide prevention coordinators who are available to assist other staff in the case of an emergency. In addition, there are national and local provider-led consultation groups for those who provide CVT services. Although some resources exist outside the VA system (eg, the national suicide hotline), it would be helpful for professional organizations or individual states to develop similar support systems in the form of networks of providers for consultation, referral, and coordinated care. These systems would allow providers to confidently offer evidence-based care to those most at risk and in need of the services.

REFERENCES

1. Hilty DM, Ferrer DC, Parish MB, et al. The effectiveness of telemental health: a 2013 review. Telemed J E Health 2013;19(6):444–54.
2. Hubley S, Lynch SB, Schneck C, et al. Review of key telepsychiatry outcomes. World Psychiatry 2016;6(2):269–82.

3. Godleski L, Cervone D, Vogel D, et al. Home telemental health implementation and outcomes using electronic messaging. J Telemed Telecare 2012;18(1):17–9.
4. Lyketsos CG, Roques C, Hovanec L, et al. Telemedicine use and the reduction of psychiatric admissions from a long-term care facility. J Geriatr Psychiatry Neurol 2001;14:76–9.
5. Pruitt LD, Luxton DD, Shore P. Additional clinical benefits of home-based telemental health treatments. Prof Psychol Res Pract 2014;45(5):340–6.
6. Gilmore AK, Ward-Ciesielski EF. Perceived risks and use of psychotherapy via telemedicine for patients at risk for suicide. J Telemed Telecare 2017;25(1):59–63.
7. Turgoose D, Ashwick R, Murphy D. Systematic review of lessons learned from delivering tele-therapy to veterans with post-traumatic stress disorder. J Telemed Telecare 2018;24(9):575–85.
8. Pruitt LD, Vuletic S, Smolenski DJ, et al. Predicting post treatment client satisfaction between behavioral activation for depression delivered either in-person or via home-based telehealth. J Telemed Telecare 2019;25(8):460–7.
9. Gros DF, Veronee K, Strachan M, et al. Managing suicidality in home based telehealth. J Telemed Telecare 2011;17(6):332–5.
10. Sorvaniemi M, Ojanen E, Santamaki O. Telepsychiatry in emergency consultations: a follow-up study of sixty patients. Telemed J E Health 2005;11:439–41.
11. Thomas CR, Miller G, Hartshorn JC, et al. Telepsychiatry program for rural victims of domestic violence. Telemed J E Health 2005;11(5):567–73.
12. D'Souza R. Improving treatment adherence and longitudinal outcomes in patients with a serious mental illness by using telemedicine. J Telemed Telecare 2002; 8(2):113–5.
13. Godleski L, Nieves JE, Darkins A, et al. VA telemental health: suicide assessment. Behav Sci Law 2008;26:271–86.
14. National Association of Social Workers, Association of Social Work Boards, Council on Social Work Education, & Clinical Social Work Association. NASW, ASWB, CSWE & CSWA standards for technology in social work practice. 2017. Available at: https://www.socialworkers.org/includes/newIncludes/homepage/PRA-BRO-33617.TechStandards_FINAL_POSTING.pdf. Accessed February 26, 2019.
15. American Psychological Association, Joint Task Force for the Development of Telepsychiatry Guidelines for Psychologists. Guidelines for the practice of telepsychology. Am Psychol 2013;68(9):791–800.
16. Shore JH, Yellowlees P, Caudill R, et al. Best practices in videoconferencing-based telemental health April 2018. Telemed J E Health 2018;24(11):827–32.
17. Ryan haight online pharmacy consumer protection act of 2008, 21 U.S.C § 802 (54).
18. H.R. 6 , 115th Cong. (2018) (enacted).
19. Department of Veterans Affairs. Authority of health care providers to practice telehealth. FR Doc. 2018–10114, Filed 5–10–18.
20. Department of Veterans Affairs & Department of Defense. VA/DOD clinical practice guideline for assessment and management of patients at risk for suicide. The Assessment and Management of Risk for Suicide Working Group, Office of Quality Safety and Value, VA, Washington DC. & Quality Management Division, United States Army MEDCOM; 2013. p. 1–190.
21. Linehan MM. Cognitive behavioural therapy of borderline personality disorder. New York: Guilford; 1993.

Review and Implementation of Self-Help and Automated Tools in Mental Health Care

Steven Chan, MD, MBA[a,b,c],*, Luming Li, MD[d],
John Torous, MD, MBI[e,f], David Gratzer, MD[g],
Peter M. Yellowlees, MBBS, MD[h]

KEYWORDS

- Education • Media • Websites • Smartphone • Chatbots • Voice assistants
- Video games • Mental health

KEY POINTS

- Self-help and automated technologies can be useful for behavioral and mental health education and interventions.
- Such technologies include interactive media, online courses, artificial intelligence–powered chatbots, voice assistants, and video games. Self-help media can include books, videos, audible media like podcasts, blog and print articles, and self-contained Internet sites. Social media, online courses, and mass-market mobile apps also can include such media.
- These technologies serve to decrease geospatial, temporal, and financial barriers.
- Implementing such technologies requires understanding patient needs, evaluating technologies, and training users appropriately.

INTRODUCTION

Asynchronous technologies power self-help and consumer-run education and dissemination in the treatment of behavioral and mental health. These technologies include interactive media, online courses, artificial intelligence–powered chatbots,

Disclosures: S. Chan reports grants from American Psychiatric Association/SAMHSA, personal fees from HealthLinkNow, North American Center for Continuing Medical Education LLC, and Guidewell Innovation.
[a] Palo Alto Veterans Affairs Health System, Palo Alto, CA, USA; [b] Division of Hospital Medicine, Clinical Informatics, University of California, San Francisco, San Francisco, CA, USA; [c] Department of Psychiatry, University of California, Davis, Davis, CA, USA; [d] Department of Psychiatry, Yale School of Medicine, Yale University, New Haven, CT, USA; [e] Beth Israel Deaconess Medical Center, Boston, MA 02115, USA; [f] Harvard University, Cambridge, MA, USA; [g] Centre for Addiction and Mental Health, University of Toronto, Toronto, ON M5T 1L8, USA; [h] Department of Psychiatry, University of California, Davis, Sacramento, CA 95817-1353, USA
* Corresponding author.
E-mail address: steven.chan@ucsf.edu

Psychiatr Clin N Am 42 (2019) 597–609
https://doi.org/10.1016/j.psc.2019.07.001
0193-953X/19/Published by Elsevier Inc.

voice assistants, and video games. These are especially prevalent in books, videos, audible media like podcasts, blog and print articles, and self-contained Internet sites. Social media, online courses, and mass-market mobile apps also can include such media. The communication between the patient and provider, whether a psychiatrist, psychologist, or psychotherapist, can be unidirectional and time-delayed. The practitioner, for instance, could record video for later viewing by a patient.

The term *automated behavioral intervention technologies* refers to Web sites with standardized information, similar to self-help books and static Webpages, and interactive Web or smartphone apps that use artificial intelligence for input and feedback. These could include computational recognition of speech, facial expression, vocal intonation, and text.

Advantages of these technologies are many: for instance, they can decrease geospatial, temporal, and financial barriers.[1] The self-help and consumer education book, e-book, and learning industry has allowed many providers to reach and educate a mainstream public audience. These are the most accessible formats, as the cost for reproducing books is minimal, as are training videos, which have jumped from video tapes to video discs to learning platforms. Educational television shows, talk radio shows, and also podcasts for the consumer audience have been created by mental health professionals to disseminate information.

Depending on how the product is structured, the consumer audience can provide feedback asynchronously, such as in the form of letters, e-mail, and voicemail. Health care privacy laws do not apply, as there is no doctor-patient relationship, although professional standards and ethics do exist and there should always be caution when providing medical advice. Finally, these technologies can flexibly adapt information for professional education.

In previous articles, we described integration of mobile apps into psychiatric treatment,[2] asynchronous technologies,[3] and guidelines for telepsychiatry.[4] In this article, we describe self-help and automated technologies: the different technologies, how to implement such technologies in existing clinical services, and how to implement according to patient needs. This category does not involve active clinician involvement, like that seen in clinical messaging apps and exposure therapy apps.

SELF-HELP AND AUTOMATED TECHNOLOGIES
Blogs and News Sites

The use of Internet Web sites can provide education and support for those with severe mental illness. In a survey of 274 patients with severe mental illness (SMI), 112 used the Internet, with a smaller rate of usage (26.8%–34.8%) for interactive media, like message boards, wikis, video visits, role-playing games, and blogs. Age and education matter: the higher the education and the lower the age, the more likely users were to use the Internet.[5]

Medical societies and scientific journals, such as *Nature,* maintain blogs that package content for both consumer audiences and professional audiences. The cost to entry ranges from low to free. Blogging as part of a wider distribution network can help bring attention of posts to a wider audience, such as joining *Psychology Today, Huffington Post*, or the American Psychiatric Association's numerous news sections, such as *Psychiatric News* and online blogs, like *Healthy Minds* and their telepsychiatry blog.[6]

Furthermore, blogs can link to and incorporate advanced features, such as questionnaires, video streaming, and audio podcasts,[6] and vice versa. The delineation between such types of content can blend together. For instance, YouTube has moved beyond distribution and storage of videos, and has incorporated social media features, including newsfeed, sharing, commenting, image distribution, and voting.[7]

Content authors can create Web sites and blogs on free services, such as Google Sites, Google's Blogspot, or their institution's own Web-hosting providers. Commercial services include Simvoly, Wix, Squarespace, and Weebly, which all have varying price structures and features. Advanced features, such as customized domain names and interactive features, often require additional payment.

Social Media

Using social media is now essential for education and advocacy and can be helpful to reduce stigma in both patients and practitioners, as well as to provide social support.[6] Twitter tweets, Facebook posts, and Instagram image uploads can boost patient advocacy efforts and disseminate both truthful and false health care information. For instance, Mental Health America's @MentalHealthAm account promotes mental health; Headspace Australia at @headspace_aus addresses youth issues; and health system departments, such as @UCSFPsychiatry and @YalePsychiatry, use social media for announcing events and accomplishments.

Professionalism and blogging guidelines have been proposed by the Federation of State Medical Boards, the American Medical Association, and the American Psychiatric Association to help guide health care practitioners wanting to work in social media. However, privacy and confidentiality can be issues, especially when one's own patient posts publicly, and providers or health systems respond to their own patient's inquiries. In such cases, it can be helpful to post nonpersonalized texts requesting the patient to contact the provider directly.

Social media can support persons with SMI.[8] A recent survey explored how social media users who self-identified as having a mental illness, reporting schizophrenia, bipolar disorder, or depression, were engaging with social media. Adults age 35 and younger were more likely to use Instagram, Snapchat, and their mobile phone to access social media. Almost all (85%) of the 135 who responded to surveys were interested in education dissemination through social media. Users used social media to connect with others, learn about mental illness from others, and share their own experiences with mental illness; they additionally expressed interest in social media about overall health topics and coping with mental health symptoms. This could be useful, as previous studies have found value for patients to learn about others' experiences with illness. However, the survey skewed to include those with high education levels and functioning, those who were non-Hispanic white, and fewer male individuals, and the results were not linked with clinical data.[9]

In a similar survey, others found that the use of Facebook and Twitter in persons with SMI in community psychiatric care mirrored that of the general population.[10] Persons with SMI turning to social media shared experiences, got advice, and supported others with similar mental health problems[11] and were interested in physical and mental health service communication through popular social media.[9]

Numerous marketing tools exist to help content authors create images, schedule posts, and reshare content. Many such tools are used by professional marketers and communication professionals to more efficiently manage content among multiple social networks, and include analytics that gauge the effectiveness of a marketing campaign. Customer support tools also can integrate with social media networks to help organizations manage users' replies and messages.

Online Courses

Patients also can opt to join free and for-pay online courses to learn more about conditions and treatments. For instance, Udemy, edX, and Coursera all offer courses on depression, anxiety, and other psychiatric conditions. The UC Berkeley Greater Good Science Center has backed courses teaching positive psychology principles to both professionals and consumers. And professors, such as Drew Ramsay at Columbia University, have created courses around nutrition and psychiatry. Traditional, established universities have generally embraced online courses and have provided electronic versions of popular courses.

Online course software can help authors structure content, grade quizzes, edit videos, and process payments. Some course hosts charge higher prices for students who wish to earn a signed certificate, and little to no fees for those auditing course content.

Mobile Apps

Apps can provide self-help and stand-alone health services, which differ from the apps and platforms previously discussed in which clinicians and health systems were either actively involved or were guiding the app's treatment. These services are akin to self-management with self-help books. This is useful because interventions can be standardized, based on scientific evidence. Users can use the app when they want, where they want, repeat content to reinforce learning, and can use multiple apps or interventions to address the issues they need.[12]

Although the advantage of these apps is their ability to reach millions of people at any moment, their scalability also presents challenges. Emerging evidence suggests that engagement with self-care apps is often lower in real world clinical use than predicted from pilot studies in which patients are offered extra support and resources.[13] And, most patients still seek and prefer face-to-face treatments over apps.[14] Much of the clinical evidence for apps for self-care are in feasibility or pilot studies.

One popular category of apps is peer support. PRIME and PRIME-D (personalized real-time intervention for motivational enhancement) addressed persons with schizophrenia and depression, respectively. These apps, developed by teams at the University of California, San Francisco, uses human coaches and peer communities in trials of patients, and led to improvements in Patient Health Questionnaire (PHQ)-9 depression scores.[15,16] PRIME particularly led to improvements in social motivation, defeatist beliefs, and self-efficacy. Commercial apps, such as *7 Cups of Tea*, are publicly available, serving as an anonymous self-help apps supported by both an automated chatbot and by trained volunteers. A study of *7 Cups of Tea* complementing postpartum depression treatment allowed the app to train lay people who experienced perinatal mood disorder with no in-person guidance or screening, who then, in turn, serve as support for newer users. The study found a medium effect size for the *7 Cups of Tea* group, versus treatment as usual,[17] although these results have yet to be replicated in an independent sample. Challenges of such apps include the need for community curation, moderation, and platform development. The National Alliance of Mental Illness (NAMI), for instance, launched a peer support app, *NAMI AIR* (Anonymous Inspiring Relatable), but in 2018, did not offer the app due to a license expiration.

Another popular category of apps is self-monitoring apps that enable patients to track their symptoms. Often known as *ecological momentary assessment* (EMA) apps, these digital tools offer the potential of quantifying the lived experience of mental illness outside of the clinic. For example, a smartphone app that offered the PHQ-9 depression screening scale to more than 8000 people around the world identified people who may be at higher risk of self-harm.[18] A more recent 2018 study highlighted the potential of EMA apps to predict mood fluctuations through combining EMA with wearable heart rate and electroencephalographic sensors.[19]

But, like with self-help apps, these survey-like EMA apps may not lead to their intended effect. In one study of substance use disorders in China, EMA was not well accepted by users, with nearly half stating they preferred face-to-face interviews instead of the app.[20] Reasons for low acceptance and engagement with the EMA app centered around privacy concerns. Other recent studies have suggested that frequent quantification of symptoms via apps may quickly become burdensome for some and even lower motivation to keep using such an app.[21] Especially as EMA apps today often now collect sensor information, such as geolocation, there is a need for both better education and perhaps even regulation about what data users are giving up and what protections are put in place for them.[22]

Meditation and mindfulness apps are yet another common category of app in the commercial marketplaces. Although the utility of these apps to offer on-demand mindfulness hold broad appeal, questions remain regarding both the quality and efficacy of these apps. Recent reviews examining these mindfulness apps have found they are often of variable quality, frequently untested, and often do not adhere to core meditation or mindfulness best practices.[23,24] Although those apps that have been studied may offer positive results in small studies, when evaluated with an appropriate control group, such as a sham app in a randomized study, the effect size and impact of these apps appears more questionable.[25] This is not to say that meditation and mindfulness apps do not work, but rather, that there is much we have yet to learn about how they work and how to use them clinically.

Interestingly, there are a variety of commercial apps that offer different properties with variable engagement and functions, such as meditation, breathing exercises, game simulation for breathing exercises, relaxing audio sounds, audio-guided meditation, and relaxing visual images. One review assessed 16 such applications according to the validated Mobile Application Rating Scale (MARS),[26] and assessed benefit within a pediatric medical setting, and distinguished 2 separate therapeutic roles:

1. *Relaxation*, or actively fostering the mind or body to enter a state of calm while focusing the mind and releasing tension, and
2. *Distraction*, passively offering a way to divert or create space for stress reduction and anxiety alleviation.

Anxiety apps are another common form of app on the commercial marketplaces. A recent meta-analysis of anxiety apps possessing clinical study featuring any control group reported a small-to-moderate positive effect for these interventions for symptoms of anxiety in comparison with control conditions. However, when looking more broadly at apps for stress, evidence suggests that although many apps claim to help users address stress, the evidence remains unclear regarding the validity or utility of these apps.[27]

There are many other categories of mental health apps. Overall, there are fewer apps and less research evidence for more specialty conditions. For example, little is known today about apps for children and adolescents with mental health conditions. In a review of 25 articles on mood-tracking apps for children and adolescents, investigators found that the apps were positively perceived, with a wide range of reported participation up to 99%, influenced by methods like payments and characteristics like IQ scores. Clinical outcomes and side effects were not rigorously covered in the research. Promising aspects included the potential to help increase emotional awareness, decreasing depressive symptoms, and help detect mental health and substance use problems (Dubad, Winsper, Meyer, Livanou, & Marwaha, 2018).

Chatbots and Voice Assistant Apps

More and more people are using voice assistants; approximately 46% of US respondents in spring 2017 have used voice assistants, and nearly a majority of users use them, in decreasing order, on a smartphone, computer, tablet, or stand-alone device.[28] Most respondents use them to make devices "hands-free"; of less importance is that it's "fun," that speaking feels more natural than typing, and that it's easier for children to use. Those who do not use voice assistants are overall not interested, do not own a voice assistant–powered device, are concerned about privacy, or believe it is too complicated.[28]

Voice assistants are becoming more pervasive. In fact, new types of "app stores" are dedicated to voice assistants that require no installation. *Google Actions*, for instance, lists all of the "apps" that can be accessed by speaking through their Google Assistant on Google Home, WearOS, Android, and Android Auto devices. SiriKit lets existing apps interface with the Siri voice assistant on iOS devices and Apple.

These apps recognize speech, convert them into text, and the app processes such text through *natural language processing* techniques. This processing allows apps to understand what the user wants and the sentiment of the user, instead of requiring users to type or click. Text-only *conversational agents*, or *chatbots*, are being actively used in other industries, like customer service, product orders, and restaurant reservations.

Numerous commercial apps also are using cognitive behavioral therapy (CBT) content, goal setting, and behavioral activation strategies to help users. In one university study, users had decreased depression and generalized anxiety screening scores (PHQ-9 and Generalized Anxiety Disorder [GAD]-7) versus an information Web site–only control group.[29] In this study, Woebot was described as a digital chatbot delivering therapy using a social media interface to supposedly address anxiety and low mood screening scores, measured by GAD-7 and PHQ-9, and incorporated automated tailoring, mental health information, and reminders to reengage. In a small sample of 70 individuals, the Woebot clinical trial showed improved depression and anxiety screening scores, although attrition rate was 17%, and the users' mental health diagnoses were not confirmed.

Beyond digital therapies, researchers have started to assess the ability of machines to respond in an artificially empathic manner, mimicking emotions, and incorporating peer support within the algorithm. This study preliminarily assessed for perceptions of empathic statements offered by an agent and created a digital environment for engagement.[30]

Early chatbots and voice agents have not implemented complete recognition of dangerous messages, such as suicidal messages, although Google Assistant and Apple Siri recognize "I want to commit suicide" and offer a phone number to crisis support hotlines.[31] This has changed more recently, as voice assistant companies have implemented more intelligent responses that now refer users to reach out for help via the National Suicide hotline.

Measurement Tools

In addition to digital applications that have consumable content, apps can function in a *passive* manner to *implicitly* track physical activity, sleep, and smartphone app usage, without users' *active* involvement or *explicit* input. These apps can later provide feedback and guidance to the user, such as encouragement to walk more steps or limit use of social media apps.

For example, one recent study assessed patients with schizophrenia carrying a digital device to detect activity level, time spent proximal to human speech, and time spent in various locations in outpatient and inpatient settings. Although the study included only 20 individuals, 9 outpatients and 11 inpatients, it highlights the potential of measuring peripheral markers of psychiatric conditions.[32]

A new research direction has been using face logging and recordings of audiovisual data to predict mental health risk and assessing for sensory detection of psychiatric illnesses.[33,34] However, these studies are still in research phase, and full application into clinical practice is still unclear. However, there is interest in having apps assist with self-ratings through features, such as facial expression analysis in bipolar disorder, along with getting advice in crises, data visualizations, and regular feedback.[35]

Video Games

Video games, studied academically under the term "serious games," have been used for a wide range of conditions, such as diabetes and nicotine use disorder. Games can encourage users to achieve goals with multiple forms of media: visually appealing graphics, sound effects, music, and a narrative storyline. Sensors, such as GPS location, can track the distance one has moved and have been used in apps to encourage running and walking. Some apps also use the camera to detect one's exercise movements, such as sit-ups and push-ups. Accelerometers can detect whether a user is dancing while a game plays music.

Augmented reality (AR) smartphone games overlay information and interactive characters in the user's environment. This can lead to users performing physical activity. AR also has been used in a variety of other scenarios, including social eye cue training in patients with autism,[36–41] stimulus exposure for animal phobias,[42] and schizophrenia education and training.[43]

More work can be done to help foster the growth of mental health apps beyond computers, as many efforts have been localized or restricted to particular platforms. For instance, the Finland-based acceptance and commitment therapy (ACT) app[44] and SPARX CBT game have had limited traction beyond the academic environment,[45,46] although SPARX has been adapted for Nunavut and Inuit populations.[47] A meta-analysis of serious games for youth yielded 9 studies with games that were available only on desktop computers.[48]

Video games are promising for psychiatric conditions. Clinical reductions in anxiety symptoms have been shown in 3 studies of games in adolescents, although, similar to other app and video game study reviews, study limitations include limited numbers of participants and issues with research design.[49] Similarly, studies have shown video games as tools to improve cognitive focus and reduce symptoms of attention deficit hyperactivity disorder (ADHD) to varying degrees.[50] A recent pilot trial showed an early proof-of-concept game called *NeuroRacer* that compared an ADHD with a non-ADHD population of 20 individuals: children having ADHD had improved attention, working memory, and inhibition measurements, whereas children without ADHD did not have measurable improvements.[51] As more video games have been developed with an aim for therapeutic benefit, some investigators have suggested a framework for assessing and implementing gaming approaches, including diligent evaluation of the game and clear intentions about its therapeutic use.[52]

IMPLEMENTING ASYNCHRONOUS TECHNOLOGIES IN THE CLINICAL SETTING

To successfully implement these technologies, practitioners and organizations must rigorously evaluate the technology's vendor, design, development, and clinical content. Then, once the technology is implemented and tested, leaders must train users, educate staff, and prepare to discuss patients' readiness and ability to use the technology. Funding the technologies can include grants from the government and research agencies, in-kind donations from the vendor, and health system operational budgets. Addressing security, privacy, and encryption will safeguard user data. Safety issues include patient suicidality, understanding local emergency resources, and setting boundaries with patients. For instance, patients must understand the lack of real-time responsiveness to asynchronous technologies.

Finding technology services and apps involves online searches, asking colleagues, use of industry analyses, and attending industry events. Online searches can include searches of existing apps on the Apple App Store, Google Play, Google Actions, and the Amazon Alexa store. However, such apps may not always be available to consumers. Some apps are provided only through enterprise deployment, whereas others are available only to scientific clinical trial populations. A recent study on top 50 app suggestions by app stores showed that only 4% had scientific support and evidence.[53]

Evaluating an app requires knowledge of its clinical, financial, and technology performance. Evaluators can use guidelines, such as the app evaluation pyramid model by the American Psychiatric Association. This model provides a rubric for evaluating the app's business model, vendor, privacy, security, evidence base, usability, accessibility, and data interoperability[54] Other evaluation efforts exist for apps[23,55–58] and for information technologies and telepsychiatry services.[59]

Importantly, evaluating the evidence base and quality of clinical information delivered is important to early adoption in clinical settings. Numerous case studies on evaluation of apps can serve as a reference point. For instance, apps do well with appropriate design, brand recognition, useable navigation, comprehensibility, and understandability.[60–62] Ensuring the app performs efficiently with no major delays will promote adoption; a case study of an EMA smartphone app ultimately was not used because the app's slow performance and cryptic interface rendered the platform unusable,[63] and another showed that technology errors and lack of staff impeded use of a new app in clinics.[64] Usability can be assessed through a variety of methods, including semistructured interviews, focus groups, workshops, and discussions informed by user-centered design principles, educational theories, and psychological theories.[65]

Planning to integrate a technology service will require hiring support staff and training providers. Having health care providers discuss the app with patients boosts patient adoption and engagement of mobile tools, and leads to lower attrition.[66–69] Providing ample time for incorporating the app in clinical encounters, viewing and interpreting data, and discussing data with patients is important, as seen in one case study in which physicians did not use the app because of a higher workload.[70] Another case study of an app's implementation efforts showed that time constraints and workload prevent app adoption.[71]

Once providers are comfortable using the new technology, providers can then *prescribe the app, demonstrate* the use of the app with their patient, and provide hands-on exercises and assignments. These assignments can highlight particular aspects of the app that are appropriate for the patient's needs. This can help reduce patient fear and anxiety, and set appropriate expectations.[44]

Finally, ensuring financial viability can sustain technology efforts. Chronic care reimbursement codes can be used[72] if the technology will be deployed and monitored. Industry-supported studies can help bolster the case for technology adoption, such as this economic cost reduction of using mobile CBT versus traditional and no CBT,[73] keeping in mind potential biases.

SUMMARY

The use of self-help and automated tools holds promise for addressing a wide variety of patient needs. Numerous efforts in using apps and media for self-care can help educate, reduce stigma and bias, and decrease barriers to care. Such tools are certainly no substitute for traditional care, and the gold standard is to have a mental health professional assess, diagnose, and treat the patient.

Despite this, these tools can help provide support for patients who have no access to care, or otherwise have limited access due to geographic or time constraints. Health care professionals benefit from not only understanding these tools, but also how to use them, evaluate for clinical applicability, and consider leading efforts to create such tools.

REFERENCES

1. Doss BD, Feinberg LK, Rothman K, et al. Using technology to enhance and expand interventions for couples and families: conceptual and methodological considerations. J Fam Psychol 2017;31(8):983–93.
2. Chan S, Godwin H, Gonzalez A, et al. Review of use and integration of mobile apps into psychiatric treatments. Curr Psychiatry Rep 2017;19(12):96.
3. Chan S, Li L, Torous J, et al. Review of use of asynchronous technologies incorporated in mental health care. Curr Psychiatry Rep 2018;20(10):85.
4. Shore JH, Yellowlees P, Caudill R, et al. Best practices in videoconferencing-based telemental health April 2018. Telemed J E Health 2018;24(11):827–32.
5. Colder Carras M, Mojtabai R, Cullen B. Beyond social media: a cross-sectional survey of other Internet and mobile phone applications in a community psychiatry population. J Psychiatr Pract 2018;24(2):127–35.
6. Peek HS, Richards M, Muir O, et al. Blogging and social media for mental health education and advocacy: a review for psychiatrists. Curr Psychiatry Rep 2015; 17(11):88.
7. McEvoy K. YouTube community goes beyond video. In: YouTube creator blogvol. 2019. Google; 2016.
8. Bartels SJ, DiMilia PR, Fortuna KL, et al. Integrated care for older adults with serious mental illness and medical comorbidity: evidence-based models and future research directions. Psychiatr Clin North Am 2018;41(1):153–64.
9. Naslund JA, Aschbrenner KA, McHugo GJ, et al. Exploring opportunities to support mental health care using social media: a survey of social media users with mental illness. Early Interv Psychiatry 2017;13(3):405–13.
10. Naslund JA, Aschbrenner KA, Bartels SJ. How people with serious mental illness use smartphones, mobile apps, and social media. Psychiatr Rehabil J 2016; 39(4):364–7.
11. Naslund J, Aschbrenner K, Marsch L, et al. The future of mental health care: peer-to-peer support and social media. Epidemiol Psychiatr Sci 2016;25(2):113–22.
12. Whiteman KL, Lohman MC, Bartels SJ. A peer- and technology-supported self-management intervention. Psychiatr Serv 2017;68(4):420.

13. March S, Day J, Ritchie G, et al. Attitudes toward e-mental health services in a community sample of adults: online survey. J Med Internet Res 2018;20(2):e59.

14. Kern A, Hong V, Song J, et al. Mental health apps in a college setting: openness, usage, and attitudes. mHealth 2018;4:20.

15. Schlosser DA, Campellone TR, Truong B, et al. Efficacy of PRIME, a mobile app intervention designed to improve motivation in young people with schizophrenia. Schizophr Bull 2018;44(5):1010–20.

16. Schlosser DA, Campellone TR, Truong B, et al. The feasibility, acceptability, and outcomes of PRIME-D: a novel mobile intervention treatment for depression. Depress Anxiety 2017;34(6):546–54.

17. Baumel A, Tinkelman A, Mathur N, et al. Digital peer-support platform (7Cups) as an adjunct treatment for women with postpartum depression: feasibility, acceptability, and preliminary efficacy study. JMIR Mhealth Uhealth 2018;6(2):e38.

18. BinDhim NF, Shaman AM, Trevena L, et al. Depression screening via a smartphone app: cross-country user characteristics and feasibility. J Am Med Inform Assoc 2015;22(1):29–34.

19. Eldar E, Roth C, Dayan P, et al. Decodability of reward learning signals predicts mood fluctuations. Curr Biol 2018;28(9):1433–9.e7.

20. Han H, Zhang JY, Hser YI, et al. Feasibility of a mobile phone app to support recovery from addiction in China: secondary analysis of a pilot study. JMIR Mhealth Uhealth 2018;6(2):e46.

21. Etkin J. The hidden cost of personal quantification. J Consum Res 2016;42(6): 967–84.

22. Armontrout J, Torous J, Fisher M, et al. Mobile mental health: navigating new rules and regulations for digital tools. Curr Psychiatry Rep 2016;18(10):91.

23. Mani M, Kavanagh DJ, Hides L, et al. Review and evaluation of mindfulness-based iPhone apps. JMIR Mhealth Uhealth 2015;3(3):e82.

24. Spijkerman MP, Pots WT, Bohlmeijer ET. Effectiveness of online mindfulness-based interventions in improving mental health: a review and meta-analysis of randomised controlled trials. Clin Psychol Rev 2016;45:102–14.

25. Noone C, Hogan MJ. A randomised active-controlled trial to examine the effects of an online mindfulness intervention on executive control, critical thinking and key thinking dispositions in a university student sample. BMC Psychol 2018; 6(1):13.

26. Weekly T, Walker N, Beck J, et al. A review of apps for calming, relaxation, and mindfulness interventions for pediatric palliative care patients. Children (Basel) 2018;5(2) [pii:E16].

27. Thornorarinsdottir H, Kessing LV, Faurholt-Jepsen M. Smartphone-based self-assessment of stress in healthy adult individuals: a systematic review. J Med Internet Res 2017;19(2):e41.

28. Olmstead K. Nearly half of Americans use digital voice assistants, mostly on their smartphones. In: Fact Tank, vol. 2018. Pew Research Center; 2017.

29. Fitzpatrick KK, Darcy A, Vierhile M. Delivering cognitive behavior therapy to young adults with symptoms of depression and anxiety using a fully automated conversational agent (Woebot): a randomized controlled trial. JMIR Ment Health 2017;4(2):e19.

30. Morris RR, Kouddous K, Kshirsagar R, et al. Towards an artificially empathic conversational agent for mental health applications: system design and user perceptions. J Med Internet Res 2018;20(6):e10148.

31. Miner AS, Milstein A, Schueller S, et al. Smartphone-based conversational agents and responses to questions about mental health, interpersonal violence, and physical health. JAMA Intern Med 2016;176(5):619–25.
32. Ben-Zeev D, Wang R, Abdullah S, et al. Mobile behavioral sensing for outpatients and inpatients with schizophrenia. Psychiatr Serv 2016;67(5):558–61.
33. Wang R, Campbell AT, Zhou X. Using opportunistic face logging from smartphone to infer mental health: challenges and future directions. Paper presented at: Adjunct Proceedings of the 2015 ACM International Joint Conference on Pervasive and Ubiquitous Computing and Proceedings of the 2015 ACM International Symposium on Wearable Computers 2015.
34. Abdullah S, Choudhury T. Sensing technologies for monitoring serious mental illnesses. IEEE MultiMedia 2018;25(1):61–75.
35. Daus H, Kislicyn N, Heuer S, et al. Disease management apps and technical assistance systems for bipolar disorder: investigating the patients point of view. J Affect Disord 2018;229:351–7.
36. Vahabzadeh A, Keshav NU, Salisbury JP, et al. Improvement of attention-deficit/hyperactivity disorder symptoms in school-aged children, adolescents, and young adults with autism via a digital smartglasses-based socioemotional coaching aid: short-term, uncontrolled pilot study. JMIR Ment Health 2018;5(2):e25.
37. Vahabzadeh A, Keshav NU, Abdus-Sabur R, et al. Improved socio-emotional and behavioral functioning in students with autism following school-based smartglasses intervention: multi-stage feasibility and controlled efficacy study. Behav Sci (Basel) 2018;8(10) [pii:E85].
38. Sahin NT, Keshav NU, Salisbury JP, et al. Second version of google glass as a wearable socio-affective aid: positive school desirability, high usability, and theoretical framework in a sample of children with autism. JMIR Hum Factors 2018; 5(1):e1.
39. Sahin NT, Keshav NU, Salisbury JP, et al. Safety and lack of negative effects of wearable augmented-reality social communication aid for children and adults with autism. J Clin Med 2018;7(8) [pii:E188].
40. Liu R, Salisbury JP, Vahabzadeh A, et al. Feasibility of an autism-focused augmented reality smartglasses system for social communication and behavioral coaching. Front Pediatr 2017;5:145.
41. Keshav NU, Salisbury JP, Vahabzadeh A, et al. Social communication coaching smartglasses: well tolerated in a diverse sample of children and adults with autism. JMIR Mhealth Uhealth 2017;5(9):e140.
42. Bras S, Soares SC, Cruz T, et al. The feasibility of an augment reality system to study the psychophysiological correlates of fear-related responses. Brain Behav 2018;8(9):e01084.
43. Silva RDC, Albuquerque SGC, Muniz AV, et al. Reducing the schizophrenia stigma: a new approach based on augmented reality. Comput Intell Neurosci 2017;2017:2721846.
44. Kaipainen K, Valkkynen P, Kilkku N. Applicability of acceptance and commitment therapy-based mobile app in depression nursing. Transl Behav Med 2017;7(2):242–53.
45. Merry SN, Stasiak K, Shepherd M, et al. The effectiveness of SPARX, a computerised self help intervention for adolescents seeking help for depression: randomised controlled non-inferiority trial. BMJ 2012;344:e2598.
46. Shepherd M, Fleming T, Lucassen M, et al. The design and relevance of a computerized gamified depression therapy program for indigenous Maori adolescents. JMIR Serious Games 2015;3(1):e1.

47. Khourochvili M, Bohr Y, Litwin L, et al. Pilot testing a computerized CBT program in a remote Arctic region: Nunavut youth and youth workers reflect on SPARX. Paper presented at: Association for Behavioral and Cognitive Therapies (ABCT) 50th Annual Convention 2016; New York City.

48. Lau HM, Smit JH, Fleming TM, et al. Serious games for mental health: are they accessible, feasible, and effective? A systematic review and meta-analysis. Front Psychiatry 2016;7:209.

49. Barnes S, Prescott J. Empirical evidence for the outcomes of therapeutic video games for adolescents with anxiety disorders: systematic review. JMIR Serious Games 2018;6(1):e3.

50. Strahler Rivero T, Herrera Nunez LM, Uehara Pires E, et al, Amodeo Bueno OF. ADHD rehabilitation through video gaming: a systematic review using Prisma guidelines of the current findings and the associated risk of bias. Front Psychiatry 2015;6:151.

51. Davis NO, Bower J, Kollins SH. Proof-of-concept study of an at-home, engaging, digital intervention for pediatric ADHD. PLoS One 2018;13(1):e0189749.

52. Kinross JM. Precision gaming for health: computer games as digital medicine. Methods 2018;151:28–33.

53. Haskins BL, Lesperance D, Gibbons P, et al. A systematic review of smartphone applications for smoking cessation. Transl Behav Med 2017;7(2):1–8.

54. American Psychiatric Association. Mental health apps 2017. Available at: https://www.psychiatry.org/psychiatrists/practice/mental-health-apps. Accessed July 4, 2017.

55. Baumel A, Faber K, Mathur N, et al. Enlight: a comprehensive quality and therapeutic potential evaluation tool for mobile and Web-based eHealth interventions. J Med Internet Res 2017;19(3):e82.

56. Stoyanov SR, Hides L, Kavanagh DJ, et al. Mobile app rating scale: a new tool for assessing the quality of health mobile apps. JMIR Mhealth Uhealth 2015; 3(1):e27.

57. Stoyanov SR, Hides L, Kavanagh DJ, et al. Development and validation of the user version of the mobile application rating scale (uMARS). JMIR Mhealth Uhealth 2016;4(2):e72.

58. Maheu MM, Nicolucci V, Pulier ML, et al. The interactive mobile app review toolkit (IMART): a clinical practice-oriented system. J Technol Behav Sci 2017;1–13.

59. Hilty DM, Chan S, Hwang T, et al. Advances in mobile mental health: opportunities and implications for the spectrum of e-mental health services. mHealth 2017;3:34.

60. Perski O, Blandford A, Ubhi HK, et al. Smokers' and drinkers' choice of smartphone applications and expectations of engagement: a think aloud and interview study. BMC Med Inform Decis Mak 2017;17(1):25.

61. Rotondi AJ, Spring MR, Hanusa BH, et al. Designing eHealth applications to reduce cognitive effort for persons with severe mental illness: page complexity, navigation simplicity, and comprehensibility. JMIR Hum Factors 2017;4(1):e1.

62. Ferron JC, Brunette MF, Geiger P, et al. Mobile phone apps for smoking cessation: quality and usability among smokers with psychosis. JMIR Hum Factors 2017;4(1):e7.

63. Westergaard RP, Genz A, Panico K, et al. Acceptability of a mobile health intervention to enhance HIV care coordination for patients with substance use disorders. Addict Sci Clin Pract 2017;12(1):11.

64. Kumar D, Tully LM, Iosif AM, et al. A mobile health platform for clinical monitoring in early psychosis: implementation in community-based outpatient early psychosis care. JMIR Ment Health 2018;5(1):e15.

65. Bevan Jones R, Thapar A, Rice F, et al. A Web-based psychoeducational intervention for adolescent depression: design and development of MoodHwb. JMIR Ment Health 2018;5(1):e13.

66. Bauer AM, Iles-Shih M, Ghomi RH, et al. Acceptability of mHealth augmentation of collaborative care: a mixed methods pilot study. Gen Hosp Psychiatry 2018; 51:22–9.

67. Christensen H, Griffiths KM, Farrer L. Adherence in Internet interventions for anxiety and depression. J Med Internet Res 2009;11(2):e13.

68. Gilbody S, Brabyn S, Lovell K, et al. Telephone-supported computerised cognitive-behavioural therapy: REEACT-2 large-scale pragmatic randomised controlled trial. Br J Psychiatry 2017;210(5):362–7.

69. Anguera JA, Jordan JT, Castaneda D, et al. Conducting a fully mobile and randomised clinical trial for depression: access, engagement and expense. BMJ Innov 2016;2(1):14–21.

70. Mares ML, Gustafson DH, Glass JE, et al. Implementing an mHealth system for substance use disorders in primary care: a mixed methods study of clinicians' initial expectations and first year experiences. BMC Med Inform Decis Mak 2016;16(1):126.

71. Diez-Canseco F, Toyama M, Ipince A, et al. Integration of a technology-based mental health screening program into routine practices of primary health care services in Peru (The Allillanchu Project): development and implementation. J Med Internet Res 2018;20(3):e100.

72. Adams SM, Rice MJ, Jones SL, et al. TeleMental health: standards, reimbursement, and interstate practice [formula: see text]. J Am Psychiatr Nurses Assoc 2018;24(4):295–305.

73. Kumar S, Jones Bell M, Juusola JL. Mobile and traditional cognitive behavioral therapy programs for generalized anxiety disorder: a cost-effectiveness analysis. PLoS One 2018;13(1):e0190554.

Assessing Cognition Outside of the Clinic
Smartphones and Sensors for Cognitive Assessment Across Diverse Psychiatric Disorders

Ryan Hays, BS, Philip Henson, MS, Hannah Wisniewski, BS, Victoria Hendel, BA, Aditya Vaidyam, MS, John Torous, MD, MBI*

KEYWORDS

- Cognition • Schizophrenia • Mental illness • Dementia • Smartphones
- Mental health

KEY POINTS

- Digital technology provides clinicians the opportunity to measure neurocognition, administer cognitive therapy, and connect with patients with serious mental illness outside of the clinic.
- Mobile devices, such as smartphones and smart watches, can gather continuous neurocognitive data in various environmental contexts, giving clinicians the ability to understand their patients' lived experiences in a more robust way.
- Hybrid technologies, such as tablets and telemedicine, can digitally administer neurocognitive assessments that were before exclusive to clinical visits; through these platforms, cognitive assessment can be scaled, adapted, and improved.
- Home devices, such as virtual reality consoles and smart-home technology, are novel platforms that have the potential to administer at-home neurocognitive therapy and to improve the lives of those with cognitive impairment.
- Many of these technologies remain at early stages in the developmental process, but with further research some of these devices may be prove useful in treating patients with SMI.

INTRODUCTION

Impaired cognition is a chief feature of schizophrenia and other mental illnesses, such as bipolar disorder, depression, anxiety, and many others.[1] Composed of several domains (eg, psychomotor processing, declarative memory, working memory, executive

Funded by: NIMH. Grant number: 1K23MH116130-02.
Disclosure Statement: The authors have nothing to disclose.
Division of Digital Psychiatry, Department of Psychiatry, Beth Israel Deaconess Medical Center, Harvard Medical School, 330 Brookline Avenue, Boston, MA 02215, USA
* Corresponding author.
E-mail address: jtorous@bidmc.harvard.edu

functioning, social, and attention, among others) mental illness can impact all or selected domains with varying severity and duration. The heterogeneity in cognitive impairment belies its toll in quality of life, functional outcomes,[2] and mortality. For example, a patient with impaired executive functioning may find difficulty in planning and decision, making employment challenging; another patient with impaired social cognition may find friendship and social support difficult; a third with impaired memory may find it difficult to adhere to their prescribed medication. Regardless of the specific domain being impaired, the high costs of care in mental illness are driven not only by direct medical costs but in a larger portion by functional impairment and the additional support necessitated by cognitive impairment.

Yet despite the burden of cognitive impairment in mental illness, its assessment and treatment remain limited. Although recent high-profile clinical studies aiming to develop medications to address cognitive impairment in depression[3] were negative, there has been more success with cognitive remediation therapy, especially for schizophrenia. But referring patients to this treatment or modifying medications to minimize cognitive impairment first requires being able to recognize and measure their symptoms. Unlike hypertension, which is easily measured and monitored, the heterogeneity of cognitive impairments and their neuropsychiatric assessment is often lengthy and requires specialized clinical training to administer. Thus, diagnosis and monitoring are a challenge especially in an era of rushed outpatient appointments where the average duration of a visit is less than the time required to even administer a cognitive assessment. Even with effective treatment, as in the case of cognitive remediation therapy, patients may often be unaware of their improvements,[4] further suggesting the need for more easily obtained cognitive biomarkers.

Although there is no simple panacea, newer digital technologies, such as smartphone, smartwatches, telehealth, and more, offer the field a novel opportunity to assess and monitor cognitive impairment in mental illnesses.[5] This is not to claim that a new sensor technology will replace the evaluation and care of a skilled physicians. Rather, these new data gathered from today's increasingly ubiquitous mobile devices can offer a means to augment assessment and bring aspects of assessment out of the clinic and into the real world, where new aspects of cognition, such as environmental interaction effects, can be measured. Although there has been substantial research on assessing cognition with mobile and wearable devices in Alzheimer disease,[6] to date there has been less focus on mental illness. This article offers a selective review and discussion of opportunities and challenges for the field in using smartphone, tablet, smart watch, telehealth, virtual reality (VR), smart-home, and video game technology to advance the understanding, monitoring, and care for those with cognitive impairment related to mental illnesses. **Fig. 1** offers a broad overview of the space and those technologies discussed in the article.

DISCUSSION
Smartphones

Smartphones offer a potential target to capture cognition outside of the clinic. This potential is derived from three facts:

1. All people, including those with mental illnesses, increasingly own smartphones.
2. The touch screens on these devices can record exact patterns of typing, taps, and swipes that may be a proxy for elements of cognition.
3. These data can be wirelessly transmitted over the Internet to central databases for analysis and interpretation.

Device Category

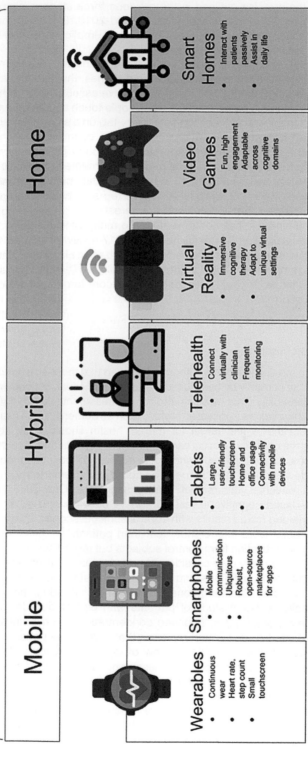

Fig. 1. The devices available for measuring cognition outside of the clinic. Devices are ordered by their mobility, with mobile devices, such as smart-phones, on the left and stationary devices, such as smart-home technology, on the right.

Although the premise outlined in the previous three steps is simple in theory, its actualization remains in nascent stages in mid-2019. Exploring this landscape in more detail, this section discusses the clinical implications and next steps for smartphone-based cognitive assessments.

As the digital divide closes and those with mental illnesses, like the rest of the global population, increasingly have access to smartphones, the high prevalence of ownership and uses offers unique potential for cognitive assessments. Although no official count exists, industry studies estimate that people touch and interact with their smartphone 2617 times per day.[7] Although not every tap on a smartphone holds clinical insights, use of a smartphone involves numerous cognitive domains ranging from attention and memory to reward processing. Although preliminary research is only just beginning to connect how these screen taps correlated to specific neurocircuitry,[8] the potential of gathering more than 2000 cognitive data points from each patient each day, at no cost, with no additional hardware (eg smartwatches), and no additional effort from patients is enough to fuel high interest.

Yet that high interest has not translated into many clinical studies that offer actual data on the actualization for mental health. A 2017 review of smartphones and cognition across numerous areas of medicine summarized the landscape then as "nascent" with "results remaining[ing] contradictory and inclusive."[9] Although this review did not focus on mental health, it did discuss the three core targets for smartphone assessment of cognition:

1. Attention
2. Memory
3. Reward processing

Relevant to mental health, the authors concluded that these smartphone cognitive assessments may currently be best suited to identify individual, not population, markers of cognitive vulnerability. That these smartphone assessments have not yielded more universal digital biomarkers in diseases states, such as dementia, or in healthy control subjects suggests that a first target for mental health should likely also be individual outcomes. In the context of clinical care and monitoring patients for cognitive side effects of medications, for example, such individual models still hold enormous potential.

To date, few studies have actually explored using smartphone assessments of cognition in patients with mental health diagnoses. One 2018 paper examined smartphone-based cognitive assessment in 34 patients with substance abuse over 1 week but yielded mixed results with control subjects scoring lower on assessments, such as the color-word interference, test than patients.[10] These results may reflect lack of effort or motivation from control subjects but regardless do underscore "cognitive capacities may vary over considerably shorter temporal intervals as a function of environmental contexts, fatigue, and other factors that fluctuate on a daily basis," and this can be captured via smartphone assessments.[10] Although not assessing cognition specifically, a recent study of patients with bipolar disorder assessed screen taps with the hypothesis that "Impaired concentration was hypothesized to manifest as increased interkey delay" and reported that screen use patterns were correlated with depression scores.[11] A 2018 review of digital technologies for assessment of cognition also covered smartphone assessments across a broad range of disorders but did not report on any mental health–specific studies.[12] Although this article does not offer a scoping review of all literature, these two studies do highlight the feasibility of smartphone-based cognitive assessment in mental health patients and the need for further research. **Fig. 2** illustrates ongoing smartphone-based cognitive assessment work from the authors' research group.

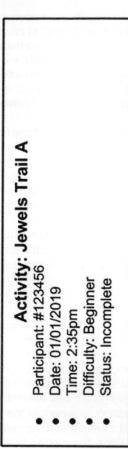

Activity: Jewels Trail A

Participant: #123456
Date: 01/01/2019
Time: 2:35pm
Difficulty: Beginner
Status: Incomplete

-
-
-
-
-

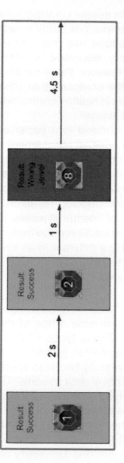

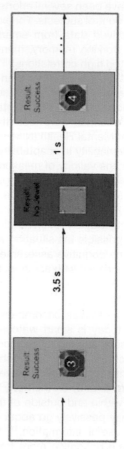

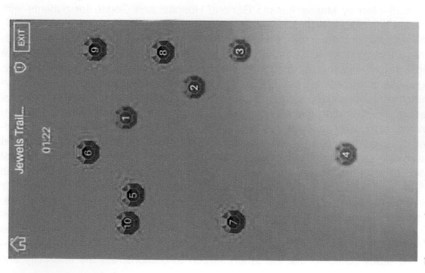

Fig. 2. A demonstration of a digital Trail Making Test on the mindLAMP app. A user is shown numbered jewels on a screen and instructed to tap the jewels in increasing chronologic order. The clinician is shown a summary of the user's taps including time taken and correct/incorrect value. (*Courtesy of Beth Israel Deaconess Medical Center, Boston, MA.*)

There have been several efforts to assess smartphone-based cognitive assessment in healthy control subjects. For example, one study assessed whether 1 week of touch screen–derived data from smartphone use may correlate with cognitive domains including working memory, memory, executive function, language, and intelligence and reported high correlations.[11] However, these results have not yet been replicated or verified by groups other than the company that created the app featured in the study. It remains unclear how results in healthy control subjects may or may not generalize to those with specific mental illness.

Core challenges were recently outlined in a paper exploring translating National Institute of Mental Health (NIMH) cognitive assessments to a mobile format.[13] These included variability in adaptability of assessments to mobile devices, device variance that threatens validity of measurements especially as related to quantifying reaction time, a need for better user engagement, and other factors. Although each of these challenges is the area of active and ongoing research, the clinical implications are that today cognitive assessment for mental illnesses is a promising research field but not yet ready for routine clinical use. Given the rapid advances in the digital health field, it is possible the situation will be different in as little as 2 years. But at this time smartphone cognitive assessments have not yet been well studied or validated for clinical use cases with actual patients.

Wearables

Although wearables encompass a diverse range of devices, the most well-known category today is smart watches. These types of devices are able to record data from sensors, such as GPS, accelerometer, gyroscope, and heart rate, and some devices, such as the Apple Watch with its two-lead electrocardiogram, are equipped with specific technology to gather novel data streams. The versatility of these sensors when worn directly on the body along with their low cost have raised new interest in their use within and outside of the clinic. Their biggest attraction, however, is that a patient may passively go about their day-to-day life and still produce and consume clinically useful information.[14] Studies using these wearables for mental health tracking are becoming more frequent: the University of California San Francisco is now using Apple's ResearchKit to study mental health in LGBTQ + individuals, and the National Institute of Mental Health recently awarded a $1.8 million grant to a study jointly conducted by Massachusetts General Hospital and Cogito for patients with depression and bipolar disorder.[14]

The measurements from wearable sensors can provide key clinical insight into factors that affect patients with mental illness, such as sleep, exercise, and more.[15] For example, kinesthetic and geospatial sensor data are used to model exercise activity, linking to exercise-mediated changes in cognition; one study was able to identify psychomotor retardation in a patient that then informed a clinical focus on subsyndromal depression.[15] Presenting this clinically relevant data to their patient as rationale for continuing or modifying their treatment plan also increased the patient's self-motivation and adherence to exercise, they note.[15] However, it was also noted that the heart rate sensor and likely other sensors were not of medical grade,[16] and that adoption of such technology in older adults would be difficult if it were not easy to use.[15] Sensor accuracy and device usability among other practical considerations remain important concerns in the exploration of wearable-based mental health care.

Smart watches, unlike other categories of wearables, come with an additional interaction modality: a diminutive but robust digital touch screen. Although most studies have relied on the translation of sensor-derived digital biomarkers into biologic correlates, one study opted to use the touch screen to demonstrate the feasibility and validity of cognitive measurements from daily surveys and validated the cognition assessments patients would interact with.[16] They found that mood was moderately correlated to clinical tests for cognition and depression.[16] In measuring usability, patients stated that tasks and assessments were easier when incorporated into their daily lifestyles via smart watches, leading to higher adherence. They noted, however, that although they had "gameified" the assessments to increase motivation, patient interaction might vary based on the severity of symptoms they experience from their mental illness, their mood on a particular day, or whether they had remembered to wear the device at all.[16] Additionally, as more general consideration, patients with visual disorders or older patients might struggle interacting with a 40-mm screen on their wrist. More research is needed to understand these usability concerns before implementing smart watch touch screen technology into widespread clinical practice.

It is clear that when correlated biologically, wearable sensors provide a low-cost and low-effort platform for clinicians to identify and quantify a wide spectrum of factors affecting cognition and Serious Mental Illness (SMI) in general. Before such devices as the Apple Watch can be used to measure cognition actively, cognitive assessments need to be redesigned to decrease patient time and effort, and adapted for smaller screens.

Tablets

Tablets provide another method of performing digital cognitive assessment in a nonclinical setting. They share this ability with smartphones, a device category that is identical in almost every way except physical and sometimes computational size; many tablets run the same operating system as their most closely related smartphones. Although tablets are universally less popular than smartphones, they are still clinically actionable devices. They attain high usage levels among certain demographics; a clinically relevant example is seen in the popularity of tablets among older persons. A study in 2018 showed that although 92% of Millennials own smartphones compared with 67% of Baby Boomers (born 1946–1964), their tablet usage rates are nearly identical, with 54% of Millennials owning tablets compared with 52% of Baby Boomers.[17] In the context of assessing cognition, studies have suggested that older patients may even prefer using tablets to paper-and-pencil methods.[18] Considering that this demographic is most vulnerable to dementia, exploring this proclivity could be an actionable route in developing engaging, widely used cognitive therapy outside of the clinic.

Aside from remaining popular in the older population, tablets belong in a unique niche of consumer electronics, because they are a hybrid of the hyperportable smartphone and the powerful, user-friendly personal computer. This niche provides tablets the opportunity to administer cognitive assessments that are traditionally administered in the clinic via paper and pencil, in a semimobile way. These cognitive assessments are often used when studying and diagnosing dementia and age-related cognitive disorders, including Alzheimer disease, which affects more than 5.7 million Americans.[19] Such apps as CogniSense can provide clinicians the ability to perform cognitive assessments with an iPad app[20]; its diagnostic performance rivals and even surpasses that of the Mini-Cog and Mini-Mental State Exam,[21] the latter of which is the most popular examination among clinicians in the diagnosis of age-related dementia.[22] However, this app, as do all other neurocognitive assessment apps, needs to be used in diverse, widespread studies to determine its true validity.[23]

Tablet-based cognitive assessment is currently available for use in SMI. One example is the Cambridge Neuropsychological Test Automated Battery,[24] an assessment that has been shown effective in identifying significant deficits across many cognitive domains,[25] such as executive function,[26] in those with schizophrenia. Another popular tablet-based examination is the Brief Assessment of Cognition in Schizophrenia (BACS), a cognitive test with the ability to distinguish patients with SMI from control subjects.[27] It has been shown that there is no significant difference in composite scores between digitally administered and paper-and-pencil BACS,[28] suggesting that the gold standard quality of the paper-and-pencil format is preserved when BACS is administered digitally. When not only comparing between the digital and analog methods but also within the digital realm, tablet-administered examinations provide similar performance to those of smartphones.[29] However, although there seems to be no significant difference in the assessment of cognition across different platforms, familiarity and comfort with tablet technology may be a source of bias in assessing cognition within the tablet platform itself, because it is suggested that individuals comfortable with iPads and other tablets may perform better in certain areas of cognitive assessment than those who are not.[30] In each of these cases, tablets are shown to provide accurate measures of cognition when compared with traditional forms of cognitive testing, although more research needs to be done to determine the bias effects of familiarity with tablet technology, age, and other potentially confounding variables.

Another benefit of tablets is that unlike paper-and-pencil examinations, which rely exclusively on clinician expertise and may vary based on setting, app-based examinations can be standardized and adapted in scalable way. A useful case of examination standardization is seen in the portability of digital cognition assessments across different languages. For example, studies have validated versions of BACS in Mandarin,[31] Japanese,[32] Brazilian Portuguese,[33] and Italian.[18] However, studies have suggested that bias exists when applying BACS across cultural-linguistic borders; one study found that applying the American norms found in BACS to Mandarin-speaking Chinese population resulted in bias with regard to several performance domains, such as verbal memory, verbal fluency, and symbol coding.[31] More research needs to be done in studying the cultural effects of assessing cognition, but with the portability and scalability of app-based cognition examinations, tablets may provide a great platform to conduct this work.

A future direction for tablet-based cognitive assessment is the development of tests that are sensitive enough to predict cognitive decline in the future. Popular screening assessments, such as the Montreal Cognitive Assessment, are effective at detecting cognitive impairment,[34] but because of their simplicity they only work after the onset of obvious cognitive symptoms. Along with smartphones, tablets can capture a wide range of passive data during a cognitive assessment, such as touch locations and time spent on each activity; these data may be useful in creating more robust cognitive assessments and examinations. In conjunction with smartphones, more research needs to be conducted to understand the ways in which testing can be administered and cognition can be measured via tablets and mobile devices in general.

Telehealth

One well-established avenue for technology-based care is telehealth, or the use of electronic information and telecommunications technologies to support and promote long-distance clinical health care. Although there are many technologies that fall under the umbrella of telehealth, one of particular interest is the use of video conferencing to provide care. Video conferencing in telemedicine has been used to conduct psychiatric interviews and consultations; help the management of medical conditions, including stroke, diabetes, cancer, depression, and post-traumatic stress disorder;

and assess a patient's neurocognition.[35] However, the effectiveness of using video conferencing to assess a patient's neurocognition is still being debated.[36]

Teleneuropsychological video conferencing aims to assess cognitive functioning in individuals via face-to-face video conference with providers. Some of the noted benefits for using this service include patient convenience and potential cost savings; reduction in interpersonal anxiety; standardized instructions to ensure consistency in delivery; and broader patient contact for less accessible populations, such as those situated in rural, urban, and culturally diverse settings.[36] Additionally, teleneuropsychological video conferencing is well received across the geriatric population, from those living in nursing homes or community-dwelling environments to those remaining in their homes under the supervision of caregivers or physicians.[37] Shortcomings of this approach include difficulty in performing hands-on portions of testing, specifically for measures requiring patients to write or draw, and challenges related to observing behavior because of poor camera angles or Internet connection quality. Consensus has not been achieved on the reliability and validity of video conference administration of remote neuropsychological testing. Although several studies have found no significant differences between the application of in-person versus remote testing, others have found differences in specific instruments within certain neuropsychological assessments, such as the Hopkins Verbal Learning Task, Clock Drawing test, and Digits Forward test. Variations in relevant study findings could be attributed to such factors as camera, sound, and display quality; inconsistency in test administration; and patient familiarity and comfort with video technology.[36] Network connection speed has also been identified as a driver in assessment discrepancy.[36] These variations are likely a barrier because of the inherent difficulty of accurately quantifying and reporting these factors.

The incipient nature of the technology and its application in clinical settings has limited literature on its application and efficacy; more research is essential to develop an empirical foundation for increased standardization in video conferencing usage and to achieve reliability in remote assessments. Continued research on teleneuropsychology will enable the analysis of its feasibility for assessing and managing a variety of disorders and support the development of general clinical best practices. The continued advancement of HIPPA-compliant technology and the introduction of reimbursement structures for its clinical applications will also create opportunities for researchers to continue advancing the modality. It will afford neuropsychologists the ability to automate and standardize computerized scoring, enabling the time-effective dissemination of assessment results within the clinical community and create a platform for the integrated analysis of findings. All of these developments underscore the potential of telehealth and how, with further research, it can be an effective tool in the treatment of SMI.

Virtual Reality

VR tasks have become increasingly popular in cognitive remediation research among those with schizophrenia. Previous studies have examined several areas of cognition using VR, including social cognition,[38,39] working and spatial memory, emotion recognition, and hallucination management.[40] There is evidence suggesting that VR methods can identify cognitive deficits in individuals with psychotic disorders.[40–42] One of the largest benefits of VR is its ability to mimic a generalized, real-life setting while actually being used in a laboratory or clinic.[40] The setting of the environment and events experiencing in the VR task is easily manipulated to adjust for various cognitive domains, level of difficult, and sensory experience. This allows for a personalized, regulated, and generalizable experience.

In addition to using VR to identify cognitive deficits, VR cognitive remediation therapy for individuals with psychotic disorders has shown promising results. Studies have shown that after completing VR interventions, adults with long-term diagnoses of schizophrenia have shown improvement in executive functioning,[43] problem solving, memory,[44] attention, and self-efficacy.[45] VR has even been shown to have similar results as Cognitive Behavioral Therapy (CBT) or in vivo exposure.[40] VR has also been widely used to improve vocational skills by mimicking interviews and job training.[45,46]

Of course, VR cognitive remediation is not without challenges. Some have reported simulator sickness after VR exposure, but newer technologies have reduced these occurrences.[40] Currently, VR research remains within a controlled laboratory setting, providing regulation of the amount and duration of VR that a user partakes in. However, as accessibility to VR begins to expand in life outside the laboratory, there are similar concerns to those for other popular consumer technologies, such as overexposure, social withdrawal, or addictive behavior.[40,47] Lastly, VR can be expensive to develop and requires high specificity around the cognitive domain of interest. This expense may limit the global accessibility of VR-based cognitive therapy, especially when smartphones, tablet, and other more practical technologies show promising potential in this field. However, such projects as Google Cardboard, which uses inexpensive cardboard to transform a smartphone into a simple VR system, offer a practical solution, and recent research suggests potential using such in patients with fear of heights. However, continued research needs to be performed on VR cognitive remediation to explore how its therapeutic potential may differ from other promising technologies.

Video Games

Video games have also been examined as a means to measure and improve cognition. Recognizing that the World Health Organization has labeled gaming disorder a mental illness in its 11th edition of its International Classification of Diseases, it is important to recognize that there is an entire research community and scientific literature devoted to improving mental health, often called serious games.[48] Serious video games have been shown to improve cognition in healthy adults,[49] especially processing speed and reaction time. However, video games as a measure of cognition across clinical conditions is still new, especially in mental health disorders. Akili Interactive[50] has designed video games aimed to improve cognition in attention-deficit/hyperactivity disorder,[51] autism spectrum disorder,[52] and major depressive disorder.[53,54] They have designed a different game for each condition that focuses on corresponding cognitive domains. The major depressive disorder games, for example, target memory and attention, whereas the autism spectrum disorder games target attention and executive functioning, and the attention deficit/hyperactivity disorder games target activation of the prefrontal cortex. Although research on the effectiveness of these games is still new, they have been found to be comparable with the current gold standard, but provide the convenience and ease of portable and enjoyable treatment.[51–53] Their research was met with high engagement rates and little dropout, suggesting that these games may provide effective treatment that participants enjoy and are willing to use. This would cause increased access to treatment, increased compliance, and decreased cost, suggesting video games have the potential to be widely used in a clinical setting. However, it is still important to consider that this increased access and compliance raises concerns regarding overuse or addictive behavior, similar to VR. This accessibility concern may be especially important in such cases as Akili Interactive, who recently stated that they are developing their own prescription, procurement, and support platform instead of forging more traditional pharmaceutical partnerships.[53] Regardless of the method of distribution, these serious games will continue to develop and present novel opportunities in the near future for measuring and improving cognition in mental illnesses.

Smart Home

In the past, many cognitive interventions and assessment tools have taken the form of assistive technologies for cognition (ATC),[55] which can access users at any point, inside or outside the home, and provide timely guidance to help individuals live more independently. One of the first uses of ATCs was in 2001, when pagers used as ATCs were shown to improve task completion in more than 140 people with memory and cognitive impairments by more than 25%.[56] A recent review has shown that since the pager study, ATCs have expanded to other technologies, cognitive domains, and patient populations, but most still focus on mobile or computer technologies and target predominantly patients with brain injury (45.1%), whereas fewer than 10% of the reviewed studies targeted a population with mental illness.[57]

Progress has been made, however, as researchers have begun to build on the ideas set forth by ATC to help individuals with schizophrenia. This development has led researchers to imagine the fully connected "smart home." In such an environment, cognition and coherence could be assessed with simple motion sensors, actimetric sensors, and switches in appliances.[58] For example, sensors could pick up on irregular wandering between rooms or abnormal movements like akathisia, whereas appliance switches could sense deficit-related risks, such as leaving the stove burner on. A similar smart-home design has been implemented and tested more recently, albeit in patients with dementia, to directly assess and even predict cognitive function based on these real-time data, such as using motion sensors to detect sleep abnormalities, which could be interpreted as an element of cognitive decline.[59] Now, researchers are taking the analysis a step further by introducing machine learning algorithms that integrate paper-and-pencil neuropsychological tests to more accurately detect changes in activity tied to cognition in people with dementia and Alzheimer disease, enabling the prediction of symptoms of cognitive decline using these smart-home tools.[60]

Although a foundation of smart-home sensor feasibility has been established, more research is required with a broader patient population, especially those with mental illness. Symptoms of cognitive decline in mental illness may not necessarily be detected by smart-home sensors in the same way as symptoms of people with dementia, Alzheimer disease, or brain injury. In addition, the feasibility of smart-home studies is much lower compared with more portable technologies, such as the smartphones and tablets described previously, but the home still represents a large portion of an individual's time and an important target for cognitive assessment. For example, passive detection of abnormalities in cognition in the home of an individual living alone could be used to alert a family member or health care provider, leading to an intervention and allowing the individual to continue living as independently as possible. The potential of smart-home ATCs has yet to be realized, especially in those with schizophrenia and other psychotic disorders, but they show promise in providing a novel way to assess and manage cognition outside of the clinic.

SUMMARY

As cognition becomes the new frontier for mental health, assessing its status and offering effective interventions will increasingly become part of routine psychiatric care. But today because the technologies to monitor and offer support remain nascent, clinicians must administer careful clinical judgment in the use of these novel digital tools. Although computerized- and tablet-based testing for cognitive impairment holds the strongest evidence today, it is critical to realize how rapidly this space is evolving. In deciding to use any of these technologies as part of routine care, a good rule of thumb may be to wait until there is at least two peer reviewed studies that offer replication of the claimed results. Most digital health pilot studies, including those on cognition in mental health, are often positive and the need for replication is critical given high probability of false-positive results in these underpowered studies. Clinicians also need to be wary of commercial claims around technology for cognition. For example, in 2016 the US Federal Trade Commission sued the brain-training company Lumosity for false marketing, and in 2019 newer startups are touting the ability to predict cognition in various mental health conditions through only smartphone touch screen interactions, such as swipes. Waiting for high-quality evidence is thus even more important before recommending use. Those seeking to make informed decisions today while the evidence is still evolving toward the level of replication can use the American Psychiatric Association's technology evaluation framework, which offers useful guidelines and considerations for selecting digital tools.

Although it is clear that digital technology holds tremendous potential in helping clinicians to understand the neurocognitive state of their patients with SMI, more research is needed to determine the efficacy of each of these devices and the useful features that each one provides. Once this is accomplished, clinicians will need to decide how to implement technology into their clinic, a nontrivial task given how diverse is the range of available technology. Some devices provide certain useful features, whereas other devices can aid in other ways; determining the optimal technological "formula" will be a challenge in improving clinical care with digital devices. Regardless, robust and adaptable methods, safe and secure platforms, and rigorous oversight, all supported by evidence-based research, will be important for clinicians when creating their "device toolbox." With this, digital technology will inevitably lead to advances in neurocognitive treatment and the treatment of mental illnesses.

REFERENCES

1. Cullen B, Smith DJ, Deary IJ, et al. The 'cognitive footprint' of psychiatric and neurological conditions: cross-sectional study in the UK Biobank cohort. Acta Psychiatr Scand 2017;135(6):593–605.
2. Mcgurk SR, Mueser KT, Xie H, et al. Cognitive enhancement treatment for people with mental illness who do not respond to supported employment: a randomized controlled trial. Am J Psychiatry 2015;172(9):852–61.
3. Mullard A. FDA rejects first cognitive claim for antidepressant. Nat Rev Drug Discov 2016;15(5):299.
4. Treichler E, Thomas M, Bismark A, et al. Divergence of subjective and performance-based cognitive gains following cognitive training in schizophrenia. Schizophr Res 2019;210:215–20.
5. Moore R, Swendsen J, Depp C. Applications for self-administered mobile cognitive assessments in clinical research: a systematic review. Int J Methods Psychiatr Res 2017;26(4):1.
6. Kourtis L, Regele O, Wright J, et al. Digital biomarkers for Alzheimer's disease: the mobile/wearable devices opportunity. NPJ Digit Med 2019;2(1) [pii:9].
7. Winnick M. Putting a finger on our phone obsession. 2017. Available at: https://blog.dscout.com/mobile-touches. Accessed March 1, 2019.
8. Huckins JF, daSilva AW, Wang R, et al. Fusing mobile phone sensing and brain imaging to assess depression in college students. Front Neurosci 2019;13:248.

9. Chein JM, Wilmer HH, Sherman LE. Smartphones and cognition: a review of research exploring the links between mobile technology habits and cognitive functioning. Front Psychol 2017;8:605.

10. Bouvard A, Dupuy M, Schweitzer P, et al. Feasibility and validity of mobile cognitive testing in patients with substance use disorders and healthy controls. Am J Addict 2018;27(7):553–6.

11. Dagum P. Digital biomarkers of cognitive function. NPJ Digit Med 2018;1(1):10.

12. Chinner A, Blane J, Lancaster C, et al. Digital technologies for the assessment of cognition: a clinical review. Evid Based Ment Health 2018;21(2):67–71.

13. Passell E, Dillon D, Baker J, et al. Digital cognitive assessment results from the TestMyBrain NIMH Research Domain Criteria (RDoC) field test battery report. 2019.

14. MHealthIntelligence. MHealth gets into the mood. 2016. Available at: https://mhealthintelligence.com/news/mhealth-gets-into-the-mood. Accessed March 1, 2019.

15. Vahia I, Sewell D. Late-life depression: a role for accelerometer technology in diagnosis and management. Am J Psychiatry 2016;173(8):763–8.

16. Cormack FK, Taptiklis N, Barnett JH, et al. High-frequency monitoring of cognition, mood and behaviour using commercially available wearable devices. Alzheimers Dement 2016;12(7):82.

17. Jingjing J. Millennials lead on some technology adoption measures, but Boomers and Gen Xers are also heavy adopters. Pew Research Center; 2018.

18. Anselmetti S, Poletti S, Ermoli E, et al. The brief assessment of cognition in schizophrenia. Normative data for the Italian population. Neurol Sci 2008;29(2):85–92.

19. Available at: https://www.alz.org/alzheimers-dementia/facts-figures. Accessed March 1, 2019.

20. Available at: http://www.questcognisense.com/. Accessed March 1, 2019.

21. Clionsky Mi, Clionsky E. Development and validation of the memory orientation screening test (MOST (TM)): a better screening test for dementia. Am J Alzheimers Dis Other Demen 2010;25(8):650–6.

22. Shulman K, Herrmann N, Brodaty H, et al. IPA survey of brief cognitive screening instruments. Int Psychogeriatr 2006;18(2):281–94.

23. Velayudhan L, Ryu SH, Raczek M, et al. Review of brief cognitive tests for patients with suspected dementia. Int Psychogeriatr 2014;26(8):1247–62.

24. Available at: http://www.cambridgecognition.com/cantab/test-batteries/schizophrenia/. Accessed March 1, 2019.

25. Levaux MN, Potvin S, Sepehry AA, et al. Computerized assessment of cognition in schizophrenia: promises and pitfalls of CANTAB. Eur Psychiatry 2007;22(2):104–15.

26. Kim HS, An YM, Kwon JS, et al. A preliminary validity study of the Cambridge Neuropsychological Test automated battery for the assessment of executive function in schizophrenia and bipolar disorder. Psychiatry Invest 2014;11(4):394–401.

27. Keefe RS, Goldberg TE, Harvey PD, et al. The brief assessment of cognition in schizophrenia: reliability, sensitivity, and comparison with a standard neurocognitive battery. Schizophr Res 2004;68(2):283–97.

28. Atkins AS, Tseng T, Vaughan A, et al. Validation of the tablet-administered Brief Assessment of Cognition (BAC App). Schizophr Res 2017;181:100–6.

29. Brodey BB, Gonzalez NL, Elkin KA, et al. Assessing the equivalence of paper, mobile phone, and tablet survey responses at a community mental health center

using equivalent halves of a 'gold-standard' depression item bank. JMIR Ment Health 2017;4(3):E36.

30. Wallace S, Donoso Brown E, Fairman A, et al. Validation of the standardized touchscreen assessment of cognition with neurotypical adults. NeuroRehabilitation 2017;40(3):411–20.

31. Wang LJ, Huang YC, Hung CF, et al. The Chinese version of the brief assessment of cognition in schizophrenia: data of a large-scale Mandarin-speaking population. Eur Psychiatry 2017;41(SS):S334.

32. Hidese S, Ota M, Matsuo J, et al. Association between the scores of the Japanese version of the Brief Assessment of Cognition in Schizophrenia and whole-brain structure in patients with chronic schizophrenia: a voxel-based morphometry and diffusion tensor imaging study. Psychiatry Clin Neurosci 2017;71(12):826–35.

33. Araújo G, De Resende C, Cardoso A, et al. Validity and reliability of the Brazilian Portuguese version of the BACS (Brief Assessment of Cognition in Schizophrenia). Clinics (Sau Paulo) 2015;70(4):278–82.

34. Nasreddine Z, Phillips N, Bédirian V, et al. The Montreal Cognitive Assessment, MoCA: a brief screening tool for mild cognitive impairment. J Am Geriatr Soc 2005;53(4):695–9.

35. Harrell KM, Wilkins SS, Connor MK, et al. Telemedicine and the evaluation of cognitive impairment: the additive value of neuropsychological assessment. J Am Med Dir Assoc 2014;15(8):600–6.

36. Brearly T, Shura W, Martindale R, et al. Neuropsychological test administration by videoconference: a systematic review and meta-analysis. Neuropsychol Rev 2017;27(2):174–86.

37. Azad, et al. 2012.

38. Rus-Calafell M, Gutiérrez-Maldonado J, Ortega-Bravo M, et al. A brief cognitive–behavioural social skills training for stabilised outpatients with schizophrenia: a preliminary study. Schizophr Res 2013;143(2):327–36.

39. Valmaggia LR, Latif L, Kempton MJ, et al. Virtual reality in the psychological treatment for mental health problems: an systematic review of recent evidence. Psychiatry Res 2016;236:189–95.

40. Rus-Calafell M, Garety P, Sason E, et al. Virtual reality in the assessment and treatment of psychosis: a systematic review of its utility, acceptability and effectiveness. Psychol Med 2018;48(3):362–91.

41. Wilkins LK, Girard TA, King J, et al. Spatial-memory deficit in schizophrenia spectrum disorders under viewpoint-independent demands in the virtual courtyard task. J Clin Exp Neuropsychol 2013;35(10):1082–93.

42. Spieker EA, Astur RS, West JT, et al. Spatial memory deficits in a virtual reality eight-arm radial maze in schizophrenia. Schizophr Res 2012;135(1–3):84–9.

43. Amado I, Brénugat-Herné L, Orriols E, et al. A serious game to improve cognitive functions in schizophrenia: a pilot study. Front Psychiatry 2016;7:64.

44. Sohn BK, Hwang JY, Park SM, et al. Developing a virtual reality-based vocational rehabilitation training program for patients with Schizophrenia. Cyberpsychol Behav Soc Netw 2016;19(11):686–91.

45. Tsang MMY, Man DWK. A virtual reality-based vocational training system (VRVTS) for people with schizophrenia in vocational rehabilitation. Schizophr Res 2013; 144(1–3):51–62.

46. Smith MJ, Fleming MF, Wright MA, et al. Virtual reality job interview training and 6-month employment outcomes for individuals with schizophrenia seeking employment. Schizophr Res 2015;166(1–3):86–91.

47. Emadary M, Metzinger TK. Real virtuality: a code of ethical conduct recommendations for good scientific practice and the consumers of VR-technology. In: Frontiers in robotics and AI, 3, vol. 3 2016.

48. Cheng V, Davenport T, Johnson D, et al. An app that incorporates gamification, mini-games, and social connection to improve men's mental health and well-being (MindMax): participatory design process. JMIR Ment Health 2018;5(4): E11068.

49. Pallavicini F, Ferrari A, Mantovani F. Video games for well-being: a systematic review on the application of computer games for cognitive and emotional training in the adult population. Front Psychol 2018;9:2127.

50. Available at: https://www.akiliinteractive.com/science-and-technology. Accessed March 1, 2019.

51. Davis NO, Bower J, Kollins SH. Proof-of-concept study of an at-home, engaging, digital intervention for pediatric ADHD. PLoS One 2018;13(1):e0189749.

52. Yerys B, Bertollo J, Kenworthy L, et al. Brief report: pilot study of a novel interactive digital treatment to improve cognitive control in children with autism spectrum disorder and co-occurring ADHD symptoms. J Autism Dev Disord 2018;49(4): 1727–37.

53. Anguera JA, Gunning FM, Areán PA. Improving late life depression and cognitive control through the use of therapeutic video game technology: a proof-of-concept randomized trial. Depress Anxiety 2017;34(6):508–17.

54. Muoio D. 2019. Akili is building its own digital therapeutic distribution platform, foregoing pharma partnerships.

55. Scherer MJ, Hart T, Kirsch N, et al. Assistive technologies for cognitive disabilities. Physicial and Rehabilitation Medicine 2005;17(3):195–215.

56. Wilson BA. Reducing everyday memory and planning problems by means of a paging system: a randomised control crossover study. J Neurol Neurosurg Psychiatry 2001;70(4):477–82.

57. Gillespie A, Best C, Oneill B. Cognitive function and assistive technology for cognition: a systematic review. J Int Neuropsychol Soc 2011;18(01):1–19.

58. Stip E, Rialle V. Environmental cognitive remediation in schizophrenia: ethical implications of "smart home" technology. Can J Psychiatry 2005;50(5):281–91.

59. Bossen AL, Kim H, Williams KN, et al. Emerging roles for telemedicine and smart technologies in dementia care. Smart Homecare Technol Telehealth 2015;3: 49–57.

60. Dawadi PN, Cook DJ, Schmitter-Edgecombe M, et al. Automated assessment of cognitive health using smart home technologies. Technol Health Care 2013;21(4): 323–43.

The Bot Will See You Now
A History and Review of Interactive Computerized Mental Health Programs

Joshua R. Moore, MD, Robert Caudill, MD*

KEYWORDS

- Chatbot • Bot • Artificial intelligence • AI • Mental health

KEY POINTS

- The goal of automating complex human activities dates to antiquity.
- The mental health field has also made use of advances in technology to assist patients in need.
- Chatbots are defined as a computer program that simulates human conversation through voice commands or text chats or both.
- The last few years have seen a significant increase in the number of health care–related chatbots available in the marketplace.
- The collaboration between AI therapists and more traditional providers of such care will only grow.

INTRODUCTION

The goal of automating complex human activities dates to antiquity. Some of the earliest ideas of artificial intelligence (AI) recorded were recorded by the ancient inhabitants of Greece. AI is defined as the study of agents that receive percepts from the environment and perform actions.[1] Homer described automated devices known as "tripods" in the "Iliad" that were assembled by the Hephaistos in service of the Gods.[2] Daedalus, the mythical craftsman, was said to have made "moving statues" among other mechanical devices. The moveable theater of Heron of Alexandria reportedly featured moving puppets. Automated machines were also described centuries later in the Arabic-speaking world. The Abu Musa brothers who lived in Baghdad in the ninth century were noted to have made many mechanical devices, including an automated flute player. Automated timekeeping devices were used in different parts of Europe starting in the twelfth century. These devices included water clocks paired to sets of bells, which were possibly used as an alarm or to play musical scores.

Disclosure Statement: The authors have nothing to disclose.
Department of Psychiatry and Behavioral Sciences, University of Louisville, School of Medicine, 401 East Chestnut Street, Suite 610, Louisville, KY 40202, USA
* Corresponding author.
E-mail address: robert.caudill@louisville.edu

Following this was the development of mechanical clock devices in several different monasteries.[3] Beginning in the eighteenth century, a significant number of calculating and automated devices were invented. Various devices were made for entertainment, such as the calculating clocks developed by Blaise Pascal and Wilhelm Shickhard. Other machines were also invented for commercial purposes, including automated weaving devices, such as the Jaquard Loom, involving the use of punch cards and which led to a transformation of the textiles industry. The British engineer and inventor, Charles Babbage, developed several innovative calculating devices in the nineteenth century, including his "Difference Engine," designed to produce numerical tables as well as his "Analytical Engine," which included a rudimentary central processing unit and memory storage, although these devices were never fully produced.[4]

In the twentieth century, major advances in processing power and the development of programming languages led to a remarkable increase in the number of applications for which computers could be used. Alan Turing, the British mathematician and scientist, was one of the earliest figures to discuss the intellectual capacities of machines. He pondered whether they could be considered to "think" and how they might be used to solve complex problems. He speculated as to how machines might "learn" and improve their own capabilities.[5] His work led to what has come to be known as the "Turing Test."[6] Scientists at the RAND Corporation in the 1950s developed perhaps the first program that could be described as using AI, "The Logic Theorist," which attempted to emulate human problem-solving skills.[7] ELIZA, a program created in the 1960s at Massachusetts Institute of Technology, used natural language to allow humans to engage in typed conversations with the program. It used techniques resembling those of a Rogerian psychotherapist. To the developer of ELIZA's surprise, many people anthropomorphized the program and developed strong emotional reactions to it. However, the program was somewhat limited in its capabilities and heavily relied on scripted responses to various queries.[8] Another program, PARRY, was designed in the 1970s by researchers at Stanford University to simulate a person suffering from schizophrenia. It is considered by some to be the first program able to pass the Turing Test because some clinicians evaluating the program were unable to distinguish it from a real patient.[9] Several significant limitations of the program were noted, however.[10]

As the twentieth century progressed, continual progress in programming capabilities led to further advancement in the capabilities of AI. The chess program, Deep Blue, was developed by IBM. It was noted for its defeat of grandmaster and chess champion Gary Kasparov in 1997 and was considered groundbreaking at the time. Deep Blue made use of increased processing power and paralleled search algorithms among other innovations to achieve success.[11] Deep learning is a type of machine learning often using artificial neural networks. This innovation led to further computing breakthroughs. Alphago developed by a subsidiary of Google was the first program able to defeat a human player at the game of Go. It accomplished this feat in 2015.[12] Other notable advances in AI include the increase of "virtual assistants," such as Siri by Apple, Alexa by Amazon, and Cortana by Microsoft, among several others.[13] These programs were designed to accomplish multiple tasks for the user, including sending messages, surfing the Internet, and providing navigation among others. They can perform these functions by use of voice command.

BOTS IN MENTAL HEALTH

The mental health field has also made use of advances in technology to assist patients in need. An example of this is the recent increase in the number of chatbots in use by patients and consumers. Chatbots are defined as a computer program that simulates human conversation through voice commands or text chats or both. Chatbot, short for chatterbot, is an AI feature that can be embedded and used through messaging applications.[14] In the mental health field, chatbots are programs that allow users to receive therapeutic or emotional support services. In some cases, they do so with limited need to interact with a human therapist or physician. These programs have seen an increase in use and popularity over the last several years. Most chatbots in use now are primarily text based and are based on PC or smartphone platforms. The United States, like many areas of the world, has a shortage of mental health care providers. Various solutions have been proposed to provide psychiatric services to those in need.[15] Chatbots are seen as 1 possible solution to help meet this demand. AI is increasingly being incorporated into the development of chatbots ("bots") that can be deployed in both clinical and nonclinical settings. A variety of proposals have been put forward regarding the use of chatbots in mental health and health care in general. Several studies have demonstrated their efficacy, and therapy services delivered via use of Internet have been shown to be as effective as face-to-face therapy in the detection and treatment of some anxiety and depressive disorders.[16–18] There is evidence suggesting that technology applications may be helpful for individuals suffering from bipolar disorder.[19] Conversational agents have been studied as a means of assisting in the screening and treatment of people suffering from posttraumatic stress disorder.[20,21] Chatbots have also proven to be effective with varying demographic groups, including youth through young adults.[22,23] They have shown promise in the assistance of geriatric patients with cognitive impairment.[24,25] These technologies can also be highly tailored for selected patient populations. A chatbot has also been designed for psychological support in a refugee population.[26] A bot offering from X2AI named Karim has been distributed in the camps of Lebanon and Jordan to provide mental health therapy to Syrian refugees. In an effort to get Karim to the refugees and aid workers, X2AI has partnered with a nongovernmental organization called Field Innovation Team, a group known for delivering technical-enabled disaster relief.[27]

Conversational agents have been discussed for use in detecting and preventing suicidal behavior.[28] Although many users of chatbots find them to be efficacious, at least 1 study has found them to be less helpful than support from peers.[29] Most chatbots are used via mobile devices or are browser based. They typically use AI to interact with users and often make strong use of cognitive behavioral therapy (CBT) principles. Chatbots are currently used to help users gain better insight about their mental health issues, including depression and anxiety, develop positive social and coping skills, and provide emotional support.

The last few years have seen a significant increase in the number of health care–related chatbots available in the marketplace. Popular media have picked up on the theme as evidenced by a *New York Times Magazine* piece in 2018.[30] Significant growth in this area is expected. One study predicted an increase in revenue for all health care chatbots amounting to $314 million by the year 2023.[31] Several startup companies have developed different chatbot programs with varying degrees of success. Some early notable examples include "Woebot," "Wysa," and "Joyable." Each of these has received coverage in mainstream news sources. "Woebot" was developed by a team at Stanford University and is currently freely available. Research published in 2017 suggested that the program was a feasible way to provide services to university students suffering from depression and anxiety.[32] "Woebot" is available via smartphone and makes use of CBT-based lessons and exercises. It also offers "mood-tracking" to improve mood symptoms and engages in text-conversation with the user.[33] "Wysa" is a smartphone-based chatbot that is also currently available for free with optional in-app purchases. It enables users to have conversations with an AI program and draws from various therapeutic modalities, including CBT and Dialectical Behavioral Therapy (DBT).[34] According to information published on their Web site, "Wysa" currently has more than 1 million users in more than 30 countries.[35] Another popular app is "Joyable." Joyable is also available for smartphones and offers structured CBT-based treatment via combination of simple phone-based activities and communication with a human "coach" via phone, text message, or e-mail for a fee.[36] Research has suggested coach-supported Internet-based treatment may hold promise for the treatment of depression.[37]

Various attempts have been made to develop criteria to assess the quality of different chatbots.[38,39] Given the large number of chatbot options available, it may be difficult for providers to make recommendations and for consumers to choose which chatbots may be most appropriate. The results of the use of some chatbots have been studied and found to efficacious in mood improvement.[40] Chatbots offer several different features, and several consumer reviews have been conducted to assess user satisfaction and efficacy.[41] Reviews assessed program features, ease of use, cost, friendliness, and perceived benefit from using the program. Reviews of different programs were mixed with some programs showing possible advantages in some areas over others.

Although many mental health chatbot programs have shown positive results and hold promise for treatment of many psychiatric problems, concerns exist regarding security of consumer information and privacy.[42] In addition, ethical questions have been raised about distribution of private consumer information to third parties for business interests as well as possible interception of information for criminal uses.[43] Ethical issues regarding attribution of responsibility in cases in which errors occur leading to patient harms have been mentioned as an area of concern. The morality of possibly deceiving consumers into believing they are interacting with a human instead of a program has been raised as another potential problem.[44] The use of chatbots and other mental health applications that use noncredentialed employees or programs that provide poor-quality therapy tools that may be ineffective or even harmful to consumers have been mentioned as another area of concern.[45]

DISCUSSION

The promise of disruptive technologies playing a role in the provision of medical care has long been discussed. Some technologies have actually lived up to this promise, although most seem to simply be a high-technology way of doing work previously done in another fashion. Telemedicine has been a wonderful innovation in the field. However, at the end of the day, apart from logistical improvements, patient care activities still require the same amounts of time. A 50-minute psychotherapy session still requires 50 minutes. AI, when applied to patient care, may offer a truly disruptive option. As noted, the software once developed is infinitely scalable. The training of skilled therapists is a time-, labor-, and monetarily-intensive process. Complex cases require a high degree of sophistication on the part of the clinician. However, common mental health conditions are found commonly, and if efficiencies can be found in the provision of care for these commonly occurring (and often clinically straightforward) conditions, great reallocations of resources could be a potential outcome. Much as primary care physicians handle most uncomplicated psychiatric conditions,[46] nuanced and sophisticated bots may come to play a role in the front-line management of uncomplicated presentations. Even cases that ultimately prove to be more complex in their management will likely benefit from the timely availability of such technology. Computer-assisted therapy is not new and has a demonstrated record of improving the effectiveness of treatment of a variety of conditions and patient groups.[47,48]

Access (or more precisely limited access) to effective mental health interventions remains a great challenge. As mentioned, telepsychiatry and other means of providing care at a distance do help with access issues, but are not significant improvements owing to the time intensive nature of the work involved. By automating some of the basic processes of acquiring basic CBT competency, therapy bots have the potential to be significant force multipliers. By reducing many of the current barriers to access, it is unimaginable that well-crafted therapy bots will not come to play a significant role in mental health in the future. Mental health concerns and questions are already one of the most frequently searched topics on Google and other search engines on the Internet. The Pew Internet and American Life Project finds that 1 in 5 Internet users has looked for mental health information, 1 in 4 has looked for health insurance information, and 1 in 3 has looked for drug information online. In all, 80% of Internet users have looked for at least 1 of 16 health topics.[49]

Certainly the collaboration between AI therapists and more traditional providers of such care will only grow. In the end, the most important goal is the reduction in preventable suffering and not specifically how this goal is achieved. An innovation that provides ready, affordable, entry-level services to the general public would appear to have a bright future.

REFERENCES

1. Russell SJ, Norvig P. Artificial Intelligence: A Modern Approach, Third Edition. Upper Saddle River, New Jersey, Prentice Hall Press, 2009. Available at: http://thuvienso.thanglong.edu.vn/handle/DHTL_123456789/4010.
2. Buchanan BG. A (very) brief history of artificial intelligence. Ai Magazine 2005; 26(4):53.
3. d'Udekem-Gevers M. Telling the long and beautiful (hi) story of automation!. In: Tatnall A, Blyth T, Johnson R, editors. Making the history of computing relevant. Berlin: Springer; 2013. p. 173–95.
4. Koetsier T. On the prehistory of programmable machines: musical automata, looms, calculators. Mech Mach Theory 2001;36(5):589–603.
5. Machinery C. Computing machinery and intelligence–AM Turing. Mind 1950; 59(236):433.
6. Turing A. Can automatic calculating machines be said to think?. In: Copeland BJ, editor. The essential turing: the ideas that gave birth to the computer age. Oxford (England): Oxford University Press; 1952. ISBN 978-0-19-825080-7.
7. Simon H. The logic theory machine–a complex information processing system. IEEE Trans Inf Theory 1956;2(3):61–79.
8. Weizenbaum J. ELIZA—a computer program for the study of natural language communication between man and machine. Commun ACM 1966;9(1):36–45.
9. Colby KM, Weber S, Hilf FD. Artificial paranoia. Artif Intell 1971;2(1):1–25.
10. Colby KM. Ten criticisms of parry. ACM SIGART Bulletin 1974;(48):5–9.
11. Tan CJ. Deep Blue: computer chess and massively parallel systems. In: Proceedings of the 9th International Conference on Supercomputing (pp. 237-239). ACM. July 3–7, 1995.
12. Silver D, Huang A, Maddison CJ, et al. Mastering the game of Go with deep neural networks and tree search. Nature 2016;529(7587):484.
13. Canbek NG, Mutlu ME. On the track of artificial intelligence: learning with intelligent personal assistants. Journal of Human Sciences 2016;13(1):592–601.
14. Chatbot. Available at: https://www.investopedia.com/terms/c/chatbot.asp. Accessed June 26, 2019.

15. Butryn T, Bryant L, Marchionni C, et al. The shortage of psychiatrists and other mental health providers: causes, current state, and potential solutions. International Journal of Academic Medicine 2017;3(1):5.
16. Roniotis A, Tsiknakis M. Detecting depression using voice signal extracted by chatbots: a feasibility study. In: Brooks AL, Brooks E, Sylla C, editors. Interactivity, game creation, design, learning, and innovation. Cham (Switzerland): Springer; 2017. p. 386–92.
17. Andersson G, Cuijpers P, Carlbring P, et al. Guided internet-based vs. face-to-face cognitive behavior therapy for psychiatric and somatic disorders: a systematic review and meta-analysis. World Psychiatry 2014;13(3):288–95.
18. Fulmer R, Joerin A, Gentile B, et al. Using psychological artificial intelligence (Tess) to relieve symptoms of depression and anxiety: randomized controlled trial. JMIR Ment Health 2018;5(4):e64.
19. Bardram JE, Frost M, Szántó K, et al. Designing mobile health technology for bipolar disorder: a field trial of the Monarca system. In Proceedings of the SIGCHI conference on human factors in computing systems (pp. 2627-2636). ACM. 2013, April.
20. Lucas GM, Rizzo A, Gratch J, et al. Reporting mental health symptoms: breaking down barriers to care with virtual human interviewers. Front Robot AI 2017;4:51.
21. Tielman M, van Meggelen M, Neerincx MA, et al. An ontology-based question system for a virtual coach assisting in trauma recollection. In: Brinkman W, Broekens J, Heylen D, editors. International conference on intelligent virtual agents. Cham (Switzerland): Springer; 2015. p. 17–27.
22. Ebert DD, Zarski AC, Christensen H, et al. Internet and computer-based cognitive behavioral therapy for anxiety and depression in youth: a meta-analysis of randomized controlled outcome trials. PLoS One 2015;10(3):e0119895.
23. Crutzen R, Peters GJY, Portugal SD, et al. An artificially intelligent chat agent that answers adolescents' questions related to sex, drugs, and alcohol: an exploratory study. J Adolesc Health 2011;48(5):514–9.
24. Yaghoubzadeh R, Kramer M, Pitsch K, et al. Virtual agents as daily assistants for elderly or cognitively impaired people. In: Aylett R, Krenn B, Pelachaud C, et al, editors. International workshop on intelligent virtual agents. Berlin: Springer; 2013. p. 79–91.
25. Razavi SZ, Schubert LK, Kane B, et al. 2019. Dialogue design and management for multi-session casual conversation with older adults. arXiv preprint arXiv:1901.06620.
26. Available at: https://www.theguardian.com/technology/2016/mar/22/karim-the-ai-delivers-psychological-support-to-syrian-refugees. Accessed February 25, 2019.
27. Jaya. Chatbots-Foot Soldiers for Mental Health. Available at: https://blog.yellowant.com/chatbots-foot-soldiers-for-mental-health-e867068b6242. Accessed June 20, 2018.
28. Martínez-Miranda J. Embodied conversational agents for the detection and prevention of suicidal behaviour: current applications and open challenges. J Med Syst 2017;41(9):135.
29. Morris RR, Kouddous K, Kshirsagar R, et al. Towards an artificially empathic conversational agent for mental health applications: system design and user perceptions. J Med Internet Res 2018;20(6):e10148.
30. Thompson C. May A.I. Help You? Intelligent Chatbots Could Automate Away Nearly All of Our Commercial Interactions – For Better or For Worse. Available at: https://www.nytimes.com/interactive/2018/11/14/tech-design-ai-chatbot.html. Accessed November 14, 2018.

31. MarketsandMarkets Research. Healthcare Chatbots Market by Component (Software, Service), Deployment Model (Cloud, On-Premise), Application (Symptom Check, Medical Assistance, Appointment Booking), End User (Patient, Healthcare Providers, Insurance Companies) – Global Forecast to 2023. Available at: https://www.marketsandmarkets.com/Market-Reports/healthcare-chatbots-market-27837519.html. Accessed August, 2018.

32. Fitzpatrick KK, Darcy A, Vierhile M. Delivering cognitive behavior therapy to young adults with symptoms of depression and anxiety using a fully automated conversational agent (Woebot): a randomized controlled trial. JMIR Ment Health 2017;4(2):e19.

33. Woebot. Website. Woebot Labs, Inc., San Francisco, California. Available at: https://woebot.io/. Accessed January 2018.

34. Inkster B, Sarda S, Subramanian V. An empathy-driven, conversational artificial intelligence agent (Wysa) for digital mental well-being: real-world data evaluation mixed-methods study. JMIR Mhealth Uhealth 2018;6(11):e12106.

35. Available at: https://www.wysa.io. Accessed February 24, 2019.

36. Available at: https://joyable.com/. Accessed February 24, 2019.

37. Schueller SM, Mohr DC. Initial field trial of a coach-supported web-based depression treatment. In Proceedings of the 9th International Conference on Pervasive Computing Technologies for Healthcare (pp. 25-28). ICST (Institute for Computer Sciences, Social-Informatics and Telecommunications Engineering). 2015, May.

38. Cameron G, Cameron D, Megaw G, et al. Best Practices for Designing Chatbots in Mental Healthcare–A Case Study on iHelpr. In Proceedings of the 32nd International BCS Human Computer Interaction Conference (p. 129). BCS Learning & Development Ltd. 2018, July.

39. Morrissey K, Kirakowski J. 'Realness' in chatbots: establishing quantifiable criteria. In: Kurosu M, editor. International conference on human-computer interaction. Berlin: Springer; 2013. p. 87–96.

40. Radziwill NM, Benton MC. 2017. Evaluating quality of chatbots and intelligent conversational agents. arXiv preprint arXiv:1704.04579.

41. Browne D, Arthur M, Slozberg M, et al. Do Mental Health Chatbots Work?. Available at: https://www.healthline.com/health/mental-health/chatbots-reviews#1. Accessed July, 2018.

42. Conway M, O'Connor D. Social media, big data, and mental health: current advances and ethical implications. Curr Opin Psychol 2016;9:77–82.

43. Bauer M, Glenn T, Monteith S, et al. Ethical perspectives on recommending digital technology for patients with mental illness. Int J Bipolar Disord 2017;5(1):6.

44. X7 Whitby B. The ethical implications of non-human agency in health care. Proceedings of MEMCA-14:(Machine ethics in the context of medical and care agents). 2014.

45. Martinez-Martin N, Kreitmair K. Ethical issues for direct-to-consumer digital psychotherapy apps: addressing accountability, data protection, and consent. JMIR Ment Health 2018;5(2):e32.

46. Olfson M. The rise of primary care physicians in the provision of us mental health care. J Health Polit Policy Law 2016;41(4):559–83.

47. Thase ME, Wright JH, Eells TD, et al. Improving the efficiency of psychotherapy for depression: computer-assisted versus standard CBT. Am J Psychiatry 2018. https://doi.org/10.1176/appi.ajp.2017.17010089.

48. Rooksby M, Elouafkaoui P, Humphris G, et al. Internet-assisted delivery of cognitive behavioural therapy (CBT) for childhood anxiety: systematic review and

meta-analysis. J Anxiety Disord 2015;29:83–92. Available at: http://www.sciencedirect.com/science/article/pii/S0887618514001728.

49. Pew Research Center Internet & Technology. Americans Search Online for Mental Health, Insurance, and Drug Information. Available at: http://www.pewinternet.org/2003/07/16/americans-search-online-for-mental-health-insurance-and-drug-information/. Accessed July, 2018.

Current Practices in Electronic Capture of Patient-Reported Outcomes for Measurement-Based Care and the Use of Patient Portals to Support Behavioral Health

Carolyn L. Turvey, PhD[a,b,*], Jan A. Lindsay, PhD[c,d],
Emily E. Chasco, PhD[e], Dawn M. Klein, MSW[a,b],
Lindsey A. Fuhrmeister, BA[a,b], Lilian N. Dindo, PhD[c,d]

KEYWORDS

- Patient portals • Patient-reported outcomes • Behavioral health
- Measurement-based care • Patient engagement • Personal health records

KEY POINTS

- Electronic health records are now capable of collecting patient-reported outcomes electronically to support measurement-based care.
- Integrating multiple features within patient portals to support patient engagement can greatly enhance mental health treatment.
- Implementation of patient portals in behavioral health settings requires specific considerations including discussing the scope of how the portal can be used by patients.
- Exploration of OpenNotes within psychiatry should expand beyond discussion of patients reading notes, and address the clinical potential of secure messaging, measurement-based care, and telemedicine, features now integrated into patient portals.

Disclosure Statement: The authors have nothing to disclose.
 ^a Department of Psychiatry, University of Iowa Roy J and Lucille A Carver College of Medicine, Iowa City, IA, USA; ^b Office of Rural Health Resource Center, Iowa City VA Health Care System, 601 Highway 6 West (152), Iowa City, IA, USA; ^c Michael E. DeBakey Veterans Affairs Medical Center, VHA Health Services Research and Development Center, 2002 Holcombe Boulevard, Houston, TX 77030, USA; ^d Center for Innovations in Quality, Effectiveness & Safety (IQuESt), Baylor College of Medicine, Department of Medicine, Section of Health Services Research (BCM 288), 2002 Holcombe Boulevard, Houston, TX 77030-3411, USA; ^e Department of Internal Medicine, University of Iowa Roy J and Lucille A Carver College of Medicine, 200 Hawkins Drive, Iowa City, IA 52242, USA
* Corresponding author. Iowa City VA Health Care System (152), 601 Highway West, Iowa City, IA 52246.
E-mail address: carolyn.turvey@va.gov

Psychiatr Clin N Am 42 (2019) 635–647
https://doi.org/10.1016/j.psc.2019.08.006
0193-953X/19/Published by Elsevier Inc.

INTRODUCTION

Mr Lewis visits his local primary care provider for an annual check-up and to discuss a recent increase in fatigue and difficulty concentrating. Before the appointment, the nurse asks Mr Lewis to complete some questionnaires using an electronic tablet while Mr Lewis is sitting in the waiting room. This clinic has built an algorithm into its electronic health record (EHR) to ensure that, once a year, patients are screened for depression using the 9-item Patient Health Questionnaire[1] (PHQ-9) administered electronically. The results of Mr Lewis' electronic assessment are made available in real time within the provider's EHR. During the medical visit, the provider tells Mr Lewis that the questionnaire indicates he may be suffering from depression. After conducting further assessment, the provider recommends that Mr Lewis start an antidepressant and Mr Lewis agrees. However, he is reluctant to do so, because he is uncertain that his fatigue and poor concentration are due to depression.

After Mr Lewis returns home, he uses his computer to log into his patient portal, which provides him electronic access to his questionnaire responses and to his provider's progress note for this visit. Patient portals are secure online Web sites that give patients convenient, 24-hour access to personal health information from anywhere with an Internet connection.[2] In reviewing how he responded to the specific items on the depression measure and reading his provider's note explaining the rationale for making this diagnosis, Mr Lewis comes to understand why his provider is treating him for depression. In addition, the patient portal contains a problem list where each problem includes a hyperlink that redirects the patient to information about the illness, including its symptoms, common treatments, and expected course. In reviewing these materials, Mr Lewis starts to recognize other symptoms he has been experiencing and concludes depression may be the accurate diagnosis. He then decides to initiate his antidepressant medication.

In the second week of treatment, Mr Lewis starts to experience an increase in headaches and nausea. He has also developed an odd rash on his neck. He sends a secure message to his provider using the portal. He and his provider correspond back and forth electronically and Mr Lewis learns that such side effects are common, but should subside. The provider sends a message to arrange a brief video visit, using a link embedded within the portal, so the provider can briefly view the rash. After doing so, the provider recommends that Mr Lewis schedule an appointment if the rash persists for 3 to 4 more days.

Mr Lewis returns to this clinic 4 times in the 6 months after initiating antidepressant treatment, and each time he completes questionnaires electronically using the tablet, including one about side-effect burden. All results are made available to the provider in real time, to the patient through the portal, and are automatically included in the progress note for each visit. During his 6-month follow-up visit, Mr Lewis and his provider review all previous questionnaire results presented in graph form in order to examine trends over time. Jointly, they agree that Mr Lewis has only partially responded to the antidepressant, but he continues to have unacceptable side-effect burden. The primary care provider submits an electronic consult to a psychiatrist within the same health care system, requesting a recommendation for a new medication. The psychiatrist refers the primary care provider to a shared decision-making tool for antidepressants, and identifies 5 possible choices for a new medication. He also recommends the provider and Mr Lewis consider psychotherapy as an option. Mr Lewis and his provider review this shared decision-making tool, which includes infographics about side effects associated with each class of antidepressants. Mr Lewis opts to try a new antidepressant with a different side-effect profile, but with comparable or superior efficacy. They also discuss whether or not Mr Lewis would benefit from psychotherapy. Mr Lewis is open to psychotherapy, but the wait-list at the local clinic is 3 months. In light of this, the primary care provider directs Mr Lewis to a link within the portal that provides access to an evidence-based fully self-guided online cognitive behavioral therapy (CBT) program.[3] Mr Lewis continues on his new medication while independently completing the online psychotherapy course. Follow-up visits reveal Mr Lewis has achieved a full remission of his depressive symptoms with reduced side-effect burden. Mr Lewis and his provider decide to continue with this integrated treatment choice.

The previously described scenario illustrates the recent convergence of 3 trends that are transforming behavioral health care and health care in general: (1) patient engagement and activation; (2) electronic capture of patient-reported outcomes integrated directly into the patients' EHR to be used for measurement-based care; and (3) patient-facing health information technology, centering around patient portals, which empowers patients by providing them access to parts of their medical record. Although each component of this scenario is currently available, electronic data capture (EDC), patient portals, shared decision-making tools, self-guided online CBT, they have yet to achieve widespread standard of care.

This article discusses general considerations and decisions to be explored when implementing electronic capture of patient-reported outcomes, patient access to mental health visit notes, and patient portals in the context of a general behavioral health clinic. It is based on the authors' implementation and evaluation of these components as well as patient activation interventions.[4–8] This is not intended to be a step-by-step technical guide to develop the comprehensive platform described in the previous scenario, and such resources are available elsewhere.[9] Rather, this article provides a discussion of implementation issues specific to behavioral health that have hindered adoption and prevented realization of the full potential of EHRs combined with patient portals.

STRATEGIES FOR INTEGRATING ELECTRONIC COLLECTION OF PATIENT-REPORTED OUTCOMES INTO MEASUREMENT-BASED CARE

In the United States, the Health Information for Economic and Clinical Health (HITECH) Act, as part of the American Recovery and Reinvestment Act of 2009, included financial incentives to promote widespread adoption of EHRs. Implementation of "mature" fully certified EHRs was guided by the Office of the National Coordinator for Health Information Technology's Meaningful Use Criteria, which outlined specific functions and features required for an organization and its individual providers to receive considerable financial incentives. For example, to meet Meaningful Use II Criteria, organizations implementing an EHR were required to provide patients a patient portal with electronic access to parts of their medical records that also allowed patients to view, download, and transmit their EHR to outside providers. Administrators, clinicians, and information technologists were often critical of the implementation of Meaningful Use Criteria, such as the complex attestation process, or increased demand on providers' time. However, this policy is responsible for the nationwide adoption of health information technologies that have the potential to revolutionize health care.

Most established EHR platforms support the collection of patient-reported outcomes, using tablets or kiosks made available after the patient has checked in and before the medical visit. Some also make these assessments available to patients days before the medical visit through the patient portal. The aim of electronic capture of patient-reported outcomes is to have standard assessments of clinical targets that the patient and provider can review together when making decisions about care, measurement-based care. Some of these assessments are required as part of the Medicare Access and CHIP Reauthorization Act of 2015 and Physician Quality Reporting System metrics such as administration of the PHQ-9, a screening measure for depression.[10–14] Over time, these assessments also may be used to inform organizational and national population health strategies by summating treatment effectiveness over entire patient populations.

There are several important decisions made when implementing the clinical processes surrounding collection of patient-reported outcomes and their integration within clinical workflow and patient portals. The following lessons learned can inform a more successful use of electronic patient-reported outcome capture. These recommendations are based on the lead authors' experiences conducting research on patient portals within the US Department of Veterans Affairs, as well as within a large academic medical center, the University of Iowa Department of Psychiatry. In addition, the University of Iowa is participating in the National Network of Depression Centers (NNDC), which has a multisite Mood Outcomes Program. The NNDC Mood Outcomes Program is conducting standardized mood disorder assessments electronically at multiple mood disorder specialty clinics nationwide.

SOME CLINICAL CONSIDERATIONS REGARDING ELECTRONIC CAPTURE OF PATIENT-REPORTED OUTCOMES

1. *Selecting the electronic measures. Just because you can collect the data, doesn't mean you should.* The first step in implementing electronic capture of patient-reported outcomes in a clinic is selecting the target clinical outcomes and the measures to assess them. Clinicians and researchers alike see the ways in which systematic electronic administration of standard measures can inform clinical care, and the potential for these data to inform quality improvement or research exploration. However, these aims must be tempered by consideration of patient burden, and the degree to which the patient benefits directly from completing an assessment. This requires consensus between stakeholders in selecting assessments that optimize clinical insight while minimizing respondent burden, a consensus that can often be difficult to achieve.

   If consensus is difficult to achieve, clinics may have a designated standard set of assessments for all patients, but allow providers to individually assign additional assessments based on clinical issues unique to a patient. Most EHRs have a feature to permit the use of this ad hoc assignment. For example, a clinic may administer the PHQ-9 to all patients at the initial visit, and at all follow-up visits for patients with a previous chart diagnosis of depression. However, if a specific patient starts to develop obsessive compulsive (OCD) symptoms comorbid with the depression, the clinician can assign a standard OCD measure in addition to the PHQ-9. Given the heterogeneity of many outpatient psychiatry clinics, implementing a standard assessment protocol combined with a system allowing clinicians to tailor assignments to specific patient needs may be the most agile system to inform clinical care. A provider may also want to assess domains that inform treatment decisions, yet are not based on a specific medical condition. For example, within psychiatry, standard assessments of side-effect burden, sleep quality, and overall functioning will directly inform treatment. These standard measures, such as the World Health Organization Disability Assessment Schedule[15] or the Pittsburgh Sleep Quality Index,[16] can reflect patients' general health across conditions and medical treatments. As such, clinicians treating the same patient, but practicing within distinct specialties (eg, family medicine, cardiology, psychiatry) can review patient trajectories on these measures to determine the overall effectiveness of a patient's medical care.

2. *Developing the electronic measures. Treat standard patient self-report measures like standard physiologic measures.* There are a range of standard measures implemented in medical care, such as the PHQ-9,[1] or the CAGE[17] (substance use screening) questionnaire. These measures have established psychometric properties associated with the specific wording of items and administration instructions. These psychometric properties are largely maintained through electronic administration.[18,19] Unfortunately, standard psychological measures are often deployed by information technology staff who are unfamiliar with psychometrics and inadvertently change wording, target time frame, or response choices. This is comparable to deploying a blood pressure cuff, and altering the calibration so readings are not accurate. It is essential to administer the published validated version of a patient report measure so the clinical interpretation is accurate and decisions based thereupon are relevant. This includes adherence to the specific language and administration instructions of the published measure. A clinician with psychometric training should review a measure encoded in an EHR before it goes live to ensure it accurately reflects the standard measure.

3. *Assignment rules. How often is too often?* Organizations can specify "assignment rules," which are then encoded within the EHR platform to signal when patients should be asked to complete pre-assigned measures. For example, a psychiatric clinic may decide that it would like all patients to complete a standard measure of depression, suicidality, and alcohol and substance use before all intake evaluations. A primary care clinic may decide that all ongoing patients should receive a PHQ-9 depression screening once a year. Clinic wishes can be encoded into the electronic health platform so that the patient's medical record flags the receptionist at check-in to provide the patient a tablet at a target visit. Most typically, assignment rules specify the type of visit (eg, initial, follow-up) and/or a target diagnostic group (all patients with *International Classification of Diseases, 10th Revision* codes of 32.* for depression) and/or a target time frame (annual screening with PHQ-9 and the CAGE). In developing assignment rules, clinics need to consider the optimal frequency of assessments. Patients may be amenable to an assessment before every psychiatric follow-up when they occur 6 weeks to 6 months apart. However, patients in psychotherapy may find weekly assessments excessive.

4. *Integrating into clinical workflow. Taking the time to do it right.*
Several studies have examined the impact of collecting patient-reported outcomes on quality and effectiveness of clinical care. Krageloh and colleagues[20] conducted a systematic review and found that collecting assessments in and of itself is not a guarantee of improved care. The only studies to demonstrate clear positive impact on outcomes were those in which the results of the assessments were made available to both patients and providers and there was a systematic workflow for them to review the results together in making decisions about treatment. Although this may seem like an obvious step, as evidenced in the review by Krageloh and colleagues,[20] some clinics do conduct assessments but have not taken the additional step of full integration, with providers reviewing results and discussing with their patients.

A common workflow is for patients to complete the assessments after checking in, but before seeing the provider. More mature EHRs will allow the provider to see patient responses in real time, and the survey results to automatically populate the visit note. This workflow requires the patient to arrive in advance of the scheduled visit to allow completion of the assessments. Given the time pressures within clinics, it is possible that patients do not complete the assessments before the provider arrives.

They can then either complete them in discussion with the provider or after the visit. However, completing the assessments after the visit obviously precludes provider and patient review of the results, although they may inform future visits.

As stated earlier, providers can assign assessments within the patient portal 24 to 48 hours before the visit to avoid time issues while in the clinic. Making assessments available through the portal may raise concerns about assessing suicidality, such as item 9 on the PHQ-9, when there cannot be an immediate clinical response. To address this, language can be included requesting the patient call a crisis line if needed, or simply administering measures that do not assess suicidality. Some have opted to use the 8-item PHQ, which omits the question about suicidal ideation. This practice is questionable, as asking all but the most critical question in behavioral health is akin to assessing cardiac symptoms but refusing to ask about chest pain because of liability concerns. Each clinic has to determine its comfort with asynchronous assessment of suicidal ideation, as well as specifying a protocol for handling positive responses.

Both of the provided examples and the recommendations are relatively simplistic as compared with the potential of large-scale collection of patient-reported outcomes combined with additional patient medical information encoded within the EHR. Several collaboratives, including the NNDC, Group Health Cooperative,[21] and Partners Healthcare Research Patient Data Registry[22] use large-scale data collection to inform "big data" analyses to improve point-of-care decision-making as well as etiologic understanding of psychiatric disorders. Barak-Corren and colleagues[22] used longitudinal EHR data to predict suicidal behavior using data spanning more than 15 years, including more than a million patients. They developed a predictive model with 33% to 45% sensitivity, and 90% to 95% specificity. More important, their model identified suicidal behavior predictors, such as fractures, wounds, and infections; in addition to the usual predictors, such as substance use and psychiatric disorders. Once EDC and analysis becomes more widespread, more complex yet accurate prediction models can be applied.

PATIENT PORTALS AS PATIENT-CENTERED HEALTH INFORMATION TECHNOLOGY HOMES

The Office of the National Coordinator for Health Information Technology defines patient portals as, "secure online Web sites that give patients convenient, 24-hour access to personal health information from anywhere with an Internet connection."[2] Typically, patient portals allow patients to view a current medication list, recent laboratory results, a problem list, allergies, and sometimes actual visit notes: the provider's narrative description of what occurred during the appointment. Patient portals often include features to support secure messaging whereby patients and providers can exchange secure electronic messages. Secure messaging is superior to "regular" e-mail or telephone because it is more secure and it allows for asynchronous communications: communication whereby both parties do not have to be present at the same time. This eliminates time-consuming phone tag.

Patient portals serve as an electronic bridge between patient and provider, home, and clinic. In the chronic disease model, patients are increasingly responsible for positive health outcomes through self-management of their illness.[23,24] Patient portals provide critical support between medical visits for patient engagement in their treatment plan and active collaboration with their health providers.

Increasingly, technical developments are expanding the capabilities of patient portals, including embedding links to enable videoconferencing via portals and using portals to collect patient-reported outcomes as described previously. Portals could also include some of the self-guided online psychotherapy programs, which have demonstrated effectiveness, particularly if coupled with intermittent clinical contact.[3] The value of including videoconferencing and self-guided therapy links within the portal is that the enhanced technical security of portals is also applied to the videoconferencing technology. It also improves usability if patients can access all ways of interacting with a health care system through a single site.

In 2017, Fraccaro and colleagues[25] conducted a systematic literature review and meta-analysis to determine actual adoption rates of portals. They estimate an overall mean adoption rate of 52% (95% confidence interval 42% and 62%). At 52%, this estimate can suggest the glass is either half full or half empty. Research supports both improved outcomes and clear evidence of user satisfaction. Patients report that electronic access to their health information helps them feel more involved in their treatment, better able to follow provider recommendations, and better able to engage in self-management behaviors, particularly for chronic diseases.[6–8,26,27] In a sample of veterans using My HealtheVet (MHV), the Department of Veterans Affairs patient portal, 80% endorsed that their portal helps them to take their medications as prescribed and 92% indicated using the portal helps them to understand their conditions better and better remember their plan of care.[6] Zhou and colleagues[28] compared portal users and nonusers among diabetic patients receiving care at Kaiser Permanente while controlling for premorbid illness severity and patient characteristics. Portal users performed better on both process and outcome measures such as HbA1c screening and blood pressure control.[26,27]

The OpenNotes project[26,27] explores patient and provider experience of sharing medical notes via a patient portal. This group compared both patient and provider experience of notes and revealed that providers were more concerned about patient misunderstanding and confusion than is warranted based on patient report. Moreover, providers underestimate patient experience of benefit from portals in terms of being prepared for visits, or understanding of health conditions. The OpenNotes project reveals patients' ability to understand the intent of portals and to use them appropriately in the broad context of their entire health care.

Patient access to their own health information also allows them to participate in coordinating their care because they can share information downloaded from portals between providers practicing within different health care systems. This is part of the expressed intent of Meaningful Use requirements that patients can download and transmit an electronic health summary.[29] Some portals provide patients the ability to send a continuity of care document from their portal to other health care systems, in the same way that providers are conducting electronic health information exchange. Federal partners in the United States, including Medicare, the Department of Veterans Affairs (VHA), the Department of Defense, and the Office of the National Coordinator for Health Information Technology have developed and promoted Blue Button as a cross platform symbol representing patient ability to electronically access their health information and download a standardized summary of recent health care, which they may share with trusted family members or providers.[30] For example, veterans seen at VHA frequently also visit providers outside this system and information sharing between VHA and community providers is often lacking.[7,31] In 2 related projects, Klein and colleagues[5] and Turvey and colleagues[8] trained veterans to use Blue Button within My HealtheVet to download a standard continuity of care document and share it with community providers. This yielded high veteran and community provider satisfaction, provider report of improved medication reconciliation, as well as a reduction of unnecessary duplicate laboratories.

Although the estimate of Fraccaro and colleagues[25] of a 52% adoption rate on average means health care systems cannot implement a quality improvement initiative that relies solely on patient portals, their electronic nature means their potential is capable of large-scale impact. Within VHA, My HealtheVet has been available to veterans since 2004 and features have been added continuously over the past decade. In 2018, MHV provided veterans the ability to download actual Dicom images of recent radiology studies. My HealtheVet currently has more than 4.7 million registered users. In February of 2019 alone, 970,000 unique MHV registrants logged into MHV, 505,000 refilled a prescription, 391,000 viewed their appointment calendar, 258,000 sent a secure message, and 154,000 used the Blue Button feature.[32] This reveals the large-scale adoption by users in the context of a large nationwide health care system.

PATIENT PORTALS AND BEHAVIORAL HEALTH: BARRIERS TO ADOPTION

The potential power of portals is enormous, yet for patients suffering from mental health disorders, the widespread implementation has been hindered by concerns about patient access to their mental health information. Mental health providers are concerned that patient access to notes would impact the therapeutic alliance and that they, the providers, would be less candid in documenting visits. Dobscha and colleagues,[33] building on the OpenNotes project, interviewed mental health providers about making mental health notes available in VHA's patient portal. Although these clinicians agreed that making notes available would help patients, 49% indicated they would be pleased if patient access to mental health notes was discontinued, and 63% stated they would purposely be less candid in their notes, knowing their patients could read them. In Sweden, OpenNotes is practiced nationally, yet allowing mental health patients to see their notes is decided on regionally. Petersson and Erlingstdottir[34,35] conducted a pre-post survey of Swedish psychiatrists in Region Skane, which is one of the first of a small number of regions in Sweden opting to make mental health notes available. Comparable to the findings of Delbanco and colleagues, these investigators report that both expected benefits and feared risks were less than anticipated once clinicians actually had experience with patient access to mental health notes.[26,27]

The OpenNotes research focuses primarily on providing patient access to their general medical and mental health information. However, patient portals have a range of functions warranting exploration to determine how best to harness this technology. Portals also support electronic secure messaging, prescription refill, appointment scheduling, and access to laboratory or pathology results. Evaluation of patient portals in mental health care needs to explore all these features.

The lead author (CLT) recently conducted an online survey with 80 mental health providers practicing in a range of organizations nationwide in the United States. The aim of the survey was to explore clinicians' experiences with patient access to mental health notes specifically and the use of secure messaging in mental health care. Although most of these providers (95%) worked at organizations that support patient portals, 67% reported their organization allows access to non–mental health notes, whereas only 38% reported their organization allows access to mental health notes.

Differential access to medical information may address some providers' concerns discussed earlier[33,35]; it conveys the message that mental health care is different from the rest of medical care, a stance that perpetuates the stigma of mental health care. At the same time, implementation of open notes within mental health should be clinically informed and address major concerns by all stakeholders. In our open-ended assessments of provider perspectives, a range of opinions supporting and detracting from patient access to mental health notes reveal some of the key clinical issues.

Perhaps one of the largest issues is the additional workload without compensation associated with secure messaging, with one provider sharing:

This has ridiculously increased our noncompensated time. We have to watch the wording so carefully because there is no nuance in written language. I think the time and anxiety around the endless e-messaging will ultimately be the major driver of when I decide to retire—right now I'm tending to think I'll do it as soon as I can.

Although uncompensated workload is a concern, the efficiency of secure messaging should be appealing to payers who could provide incentive for secure messaging. To date, VHA provides workload credit for secure messaging and the Centers for Medicare and Medicaid Services is currently considering compensation models.[36] Moreover, other providers in the survey viewed secure messaging in a more positive light. For example, one provider stated:

Most of my patients are very pleased with the ability to use secure messaging to reach me, and I love the fact that their (and my) messages go into the chart when they are made via secure messaging. This is much easier than documenting a phone call or pasting an e-mail message into the chart. There is documented evidence that I have responded to their queries and they to mine.

Many use messaging to efficiently communicate without playing phone tag and the automatic inclusion in the EHR also improves efficiency.

Another major concern is the degree to which providers can be truly candid in medical documentation with open notes. One provider stated:

It's not a great idea to have patients have full access to the narrative of their notes. I have known providers to not add diagnoses to their notes or to change their behavioral observations sections out of fear of their patients (e.g., those with significant disturbances and/or personality disorders).

This concern raises an important issue around the multiple functions of the EHR. The health record serves as a historical record, a communication tool between providers and, in the advent of patient portals, a communication tool with patients. The concern expressed reveals how patient access to notes may limit the effectiveness of the EHR as a provider-to-provider communication tool. In addition to concerns about patients with poor insight into their illness, providers also may want to communicate privately about suspicions of violent behavior risk, physical or sexual abuse, or substance use disorders. Currently available EHR platforms realize this clinical need and now provide features allowing for time-limited clinician-to-clinician electronic communication that is not included in the data fields available through the patient portal.

Providers surveyed in the Agency for Healthcare Research and Quality study also highlighted the importance of conveying the appropriate scope of messages to patients.

I work for the VA and patients use secure messaging quite a bit. I do a fair amount of educating regarding what is appropriate and I have a low threshold for telling patients if something is too complex to manage over secure messaging but we can have a phone appointment.

This provider stresses the need for structure and communication around patient portals and secure messaging usage. Like any new technology, portals are neither inherently harmful nor beneficial. Their potential lies in the ability of the provider to collaborate with the patient on using the tool to meet the mutually agreed on goals of treatment.

IMPLEMENTATION OF PATIENT PORTALS: PUTTING THE HORSE BEFORE THE CART

Within the United States, the implementation of EHRs and patient portals occurred due to the HITECH and Meaningful Use incentives. They became widespread in response to national-level policy. Implementation was often haphazard without specific clinical recommendations or policies to guide clinical adoption. In retrospect, the cart was put before the horse. As one example, in our interviews with providers about their experiences with patient portals in mental health care, many reported they first learned patients could read their visit notes from the patients themselves during the medical visit, not from clinic leadership. However, despite this haphazard beginning, today we have enough experience to present recommendations to improve the overall integration of these technologies into mental health care.

The investigators exploring OpenNotes in the context of mental health care argue for releasing notes, but make clear recommendations about providing clinical context for this practice. With VHA, Pisciotta and colleagues[37] recommend writing notes that maintain the therapeutic relationship, communicating with patients about their notes, and using clinical notes as a patient resource to enhance care. Dobscha and colleagues[38] have developed and validated an online educational program for mental health clinicians conveying best practices in enhanced care through patient portals and open notes. This training includes recommendations about navigating complex clinical scenarios and addresses common concerns about OpenNotes. Participation in the course resulted in clinician reduction in worry about negative consequences of open notes and improvement in perceived ability to communicate with and educate patients about access to their health information.

More research is needed on optimal design and implementation of this patient-facing technology. To date, much of the research has focused specifically on patient access to the visit note, yet patient portals support a wide range of functions, many with critical interactive features, such as appointment scheduling and prescription refill, all of which can directly benefit mental health patients. Operations within the VHA have developed an account activity log for 163 unique activities available to all patients through My HealtheVet. Between its inception in 2004 and February 2019, veterans surpassed the one billionth mark for total activities completed. Notably, the most frequent activities were prescription refill and laboratory results review, not reading visit notes.

SUMMARY

This article presents the potential of electronic capture of patient-reported outcomes for measurement-based care within a multifunctional patient portal. As patients have a right to their full medical record, continuing to hinder electronic access to mental health notes seems shortsighted, especially in light of available training programs to promote optimal implementation of mental health open notes. Moreover, it will delay progression to a comprehensive patient-centered health information technology home able to support fuller patient engagement both in clinic and at home, a tool currently available to patients with other medical conditions, such as cardiac illness or diabetes. The discussion about patient portals in mental health also needs to expand beyond the focus on access to provider notes. Portals support a wide range of functions, and each can be harnessed to improve the lives of our patients. In light of the increasing public health burden of psychiatric disorders coupled with a growing provider shortage, the behavioral health field cannot afford to leave such a valuable tool on the table.

ACKNOWLEDGMENTS

The work reported here was supported by the Veterans Health Administration (VHA) Office of Rural Health, VHA Health Services Research and Development Service through the Comprehensive Access and Delivery Research and Evaluation (CADRE) Center, Iowa City Iowa and the Center for Innovations in Quality, Effectiveness and Safety (#CIN 13-413), Houston, Texas, Virtual Specialty Care QUERI Program: Implementing and Evaluating Technology Facilitated Clinical Interventions to Improve Access to High Quality Specialty Care for Rural Veterans (QUE 15-2821), Seattle, WA, and Iowa City, IA, the Department of Health and Human Services, Agency for Healthcare Research and Quality, Health Services Research and Development (R21HS025785-01). This work was made possible, in part, by a research collaboration supported by the National Network of Depression Centers (NNDC), an interdependent consortium of academic depression centers. The views expressed in this article are those of the authors and do not necessarily represent the views of the Department of Veterans Affairs.

REFERENCES

1. Kroenke K, Spitzer RL, Williams JB. The PHQ-9: validity of a brief depression severity measure. J Gen Intern Med 2001;16(9):606–13.
2. What is a Patient Portal?. Available at: https://www.healthit.gov/faq/what-patient-portal. Accessed March 25, 2019.
3. Donker T, Bennett K, Bennett A, et al. Internet-delivered interpersonal psychotherapy versus Internet-delivered cognitive behavioral therapy for adults with depressive symptoms: randomized controlled noninferiority trial. J Med Internet Res 2013;15(5):e82.
4. Klein DM, Fix GM, Hogan TP, et al. Use of the blue button online tool for sharing health information: qualitative interviews with patients and providers. J Med Internet Res 2015;17(8):e199.
5. Klein DM, Pham K, Samy L, et al. The veteran-initiated electronic care coordination: a multisite initiative to promote and evaluate consumer-mediated health information exchange. Telemed J E Health 2017;23(4):264–72.
6. Nazi KM, Turvey CL, Klein DM, et al. A decade of veteran voices: examining patient portal enhancements through the lens of user-centered design. J Med Internet Res 2018;20(7):e10413.
7. Turvey C, Klein D, Fix G, et al. Blue Button use by patients to access and share health record information using the Department of Veterans Affairs' online patient portal. J Am Med Inform Assoc 2014;21(4):657–63.
8. Turvey CL, Klein DM, Witry M, et al. Patient education for consumer-mediated HIE. A pilot randomized controlled trial of the Department of Veterans Affairs Blue Button. Appl Clin Inform 2016;7(3):765–76.
9. Snyder C, Wu AW. Users' Guide to Integrating Patient-Reported Outcomes in Electronic Health Records 2017. Available at: http://www.pcori.org/document/users-guide-integrating-patient-reported-outcomeselectronic-health-records.
10. Hirsch JA, Leslie-Mazwi TM, Nicola GN, et al. PQRS and the MACRA: value-based payments have moved from concept to reality. AJNR Am J Neuroradiol 2016;37(12):2195–200.

11. Krittanawong C. MACRA in the era of big data: implications for clinical practice. Int J Cardiol 2018;260:226–7.
12. McLaughlin DB. MACRA: an overview and implications. healthcare is taking the next step on the long road to value-based purchasing. Healthc Exec 2017; 32(3):56, 58-59.
13. Russo AM. Performance measurement in the MACRA era. Circulation 2019; 139(7):847–9.
14. Walsh MN. MACRA is a law: practice transformation is the goal. J Am Coll Cardiol 2017;70(8):1096–8.
15. Garin O, Ayuso-Mateos JL, Almansa J, et al. Validation of the "World Health Organization disability assessment schedule, WHODAS-2" in patients with chronic diseases. Health Qual Life Outcomes 2010;8:51.
16. Buysse DJ, Reynolds CF 3rd, Monk TH, et al. The Pittsburgh Sleep Quality Index: a new instrument for psychiatric practice and research. Psychiatry Res 1989; 28(2):193–213.
17. Brown RL, Rounds LA. Conjoint screening questionnaires for alcohol and other drug abuse: criterion validity in a primary care practice. Wis Med J 1995;94(3): 135–40.
18. Brock RL, Barry RA, Lawrence E, et al. Internet administration of paper-and-pencil questionnaires used in couple research: assessing psychometric equivalence. Assessment 2012;19(2):226–42.
19. Buchanan T, Smith JL. Research on the Internet: validation of a world-wide web mediated personality scale. Behav Res Methods Instrum Comput 1999;31(4): 565–71.
20. Krageloh CU, Czuba KJ, Billington DR, et al. Using feedback from patient-reported outcome measures in mental health services: a scoping study and typology. Psychiatr Serv 2015;66(3):224–41.
21. Simon GE, Beck A, Rossom R, et al. Population-based outreach versus care as usual to prevent suicide attempt: study protocol for a randomized controlled trial. Trials 2016;17(1):452.
22. Barak-Corren Y, Castro VM, Javitt S, et al. Predicting suicidal behavior from longitudinal electronic health records. Am J Psychiatry 2017;174(2):154–62.
23. Bodenheimer T, Wagner EH, Grumbach K. Improving primary care for patients with chronic illness: the chronic care model, Part 2. JAMA 2002;288(15):1909–14.
24. Bodenheimer T, Wagner EH, Grumbach K. Improving primary care for patients with chronic illness. JAMA 2002;288(14):1775–9.
25. Fraccaro P, Vigo M, Balatsoukas P, et al. Patient portal adoption rates: a systematic literature review and meta-analysis. Stud Health Technol Inform 2017;245: 79–83.
26. Delbanco T, Walker J, Bell SK, et al. Inviting patients to read their doctors' notes: a quasi-experimental study and a look ahead. Ann Intern Med 2012;157(7):461–70.
27. Delbanco T, Walker J, Darer JD, et al. Open notes: doctors and patients signing on. Ann Intern Med 2010;153(2):121–5.
28. Zhou YY, Kanter MH, Wang JJ, et al. Improved quality at Kaiser Permanente through e-mail between physicians and patients. Health Aff (Millwood) 2010; 29(7):1370–5.
29. DeSalvo KB, Mertz K. Broadening the view of interoperability to include person-centeredness. J Gen Intern Med 2015;30(Suppl 1):S1–2.
30. Medicare's Blue Button and Blue Button 2.0. Available at: https://www.medicare.gov/manage-your-health/medicares-blue-button-blue-button-20. Accessed March 25, 2019.

31. Charlton ME, Mengeling MA, Schlichting JA, et al. Veteran use of health care systems in rural states: comparing VA and non-VA health care use among privately insured veterans under age 65. J Rural Health 2016;32(4):407–17.
32. Cadwallader M. Department of Veterans Affairs Office of Connected Care Clinical Advisory Board Briefing: My HealtheVet Statistical Overview. 2019.
33. Dobscha SK, Denneson LM, Jacobson LE, et al. VA mental health clinician experiences and attitudes toward OpenNotes. Gen Hosp Psychiatry 2016;38:89–93.
34. Petersson L, Erlingsdottir G. Open notes in Swedish psychiatric care (part 2): survey among psychiatric care professionals. JMIR Ment Health 2018;5(2):e10521.
35. Petersson L, Erlingsdottir G. Open notes in Swedish psychiatric care (part 1): survey among psychiatric care professionals. JMIR Ment Health 2018;5(1):e11.
36. Stage 3 Program Requirements for Eligible Hospitals. Available at: https://www.cms.gov/Regulations-and-Guidance/Legislation/EHRIncentivePrograms/Stage3_RequieEH.html. Accessed March 30, 2019.
37. Pisciotta M, Denneson LM, Williams HB, et al. Providing mental health care in the context of online mental health notes: advice from patients and mental health clinicians. J Ment Health 2019;28(1):64–70.
38. Dobscha SK, Kenyon EA, Pisciotta MK, et al. Impacts of a web-based course on mental health clinicians' attitudes and communication behaviors related to use of OpenNotes. Psychiatr Serv 2019;70(6):474–9.

A Guide for the 21st Century Psychiatrist to Managing Your Online Reputation, Your Privacy, and Professional Use of Social Media

John Luo, MD

KEYWORDS

- Online professional reputation • Privacy • Professional social media use

KEY POINTS

- Online content about providers will influence your professional reputation.
- Physician rating sites will increasingly play a role in future self-referrals by prospective patients.
- In social media, the boundaries of professional and personal matters are blurry, creating privacy risks and boundary issues.
- Providers should be aware of personal information exposure unearthed by people search engines.
- Maintenance of privacy online is an active process that requires using settings on Web sites and appropriate tools.

INTRODUCTION

Many readers have read somewhere that the Internet was initially developed for the military. The ARPANET (Advanced Research Projects Agency Network) was created in the 1960s with the goal of delivering electronic messages in a network with the ability to do so in case one of the network nodes became compromised.[1,2] Although this design may be an oversimplification of the goal for the telecommunication control protocol/Internet protocol (IP), along with HTML, these are some of the foundational underpinning Internet technologies for the distribution of information. The developers of these technologies probably did not imagine the growth and transformation of the

Disclosure Statement: The author has nothing to disclose.
University of California Riverside School of Medicine, 14350 Meridian Parkway, Riverside, CA 92508, USA
E-mail address: johnluo@medsch.ucr.edu
twitter: @jsluo (J.L.)

Psychiatr Clin N Am 42 (2019) 649–658
https://doi.org/10.1016/j.psc.2019.08.011

psych.theclinics.com

Internet with its constantly evolving storage and transmission of varied types of information.

Today, the Internet has dramatically changed how people access, receive, and interact with information. Almost gone are the days whereby printed materials, such as telephone books, maps, travel guides, and novels, were used exclusively, and these items will be soon added to the endangered species list. It is almost unimaginable that physical items, such as books, compact discs, and DVD (digital video discs), will disappear from daily life, but already some resources, such as the *Encyclopedia Britannica*, are no longer available in print form.[1]

In a related way, how patients find health care providers as well as what they know about them has changed along with the development of the Internet. In the not so distant past, people would find a doctor in a telephone book, perhaps from an advertisement in the newspaper or magazine, or more likely, from a verbal referral from a friend, coworker, or someone in the health care field. The direct referral still is the best match opportunity for patients based on direct experience of the referring resource as a patient, patient relative, or colleague of the health care provider. However, many prospective patients nowadays turn to the Internet to find their doctor just like how they buy or search for information on apparel, other goods, and services online.

There are guides on how to find a doctor online, such as the one provided by the American Medical Association Doctor Finder.[3] It provides basic information, such as medical school, residency program, board certification, and practice type. *US News and World Report* also has an article on finding a primary care doctor, which emphasizes use of the specialty organization to find a board-certified provider that is in the insurance network.[4] Patients are recommended to visit the primary care provider to see if there is a fit in terms of values and concern for your health. Nowadays, patients just turn to information online to decide whether to make an appointment with a new doctor.

YOUR ONLINE REPUTATION

Once a patient finds a provider's name on the insurance panel, their next step is to search for more information online using an Internet search engine. Anything and everything that is available online is fair game for interpretation and implication on one's reputation. Whether it is a YouTube video, picture, LinkedIn page, or a practice Web site, all content online plays a role in what people think about one's reputation. Even shopping sites, such as Amazon.com, can reveal your profile, which includes information about you, such as gifts you desire, your home city, and date of birth. Although some of this information may appear to be innocuous, it is difficult to control what a prospective patient thinks about one's hobbies, reading interests, or pictures on vacation and how these influence their analysis of how good a doctor one may be.

However, most of the top search hits on search engines deliver professional information. The search engines have algorithms that have determined that a search including the terms "MD" or "DR." is most likely searching for information about a health professional. Medical practice Web sites and faculty appointment Web pages typically are listed in the "top-ten" findings, but physician rating sites are now dominating the search findings. The reasons for the high search placement of rating sites include the assumption that these searches are generated by potential patients as well as the "pay for placement" of the rating sites to generate more traffic and hence advertisement revenue.

Physician rating sites are exactly what one would imagine them to be. The sites allow individuals to review their physician and express their opinion about them and the care that they have received. Many of these Web sites list background information, such as where the physician trained (eg, medical school, hospital affiliations, board certifications) and what insurance plans are accepted. Some of this information comes from the American Medical Association, whereas other information comes from partner Web sites, such as Doximity.com. The site Healthgrades.com provides a background check that includes disciplinary actions, malpractice claims, and board actions. It does not take much imagination to figure out that physician rating sites provide extensive and relevant information about a health provider and have become the keystone to one's reputation online.

Many of these physician rating sites use various metrics to rate the physician. Most prominent is an overall rating, typically out of 5 stars. Other rating elements include wait time, promptness, bedside manner, ease to make an appointment, staff friendliness, medical knowledge, how much time spent in the appointment, and accuracy of diagnosis. More significantly, an open comments section provides a platform for patients to state whatever they wish. Some sites allow anyone to rate and post comments while remaining anonymous, whereas other sites require a valid e-mail address to post reviews.

The implications of these reviews are obvious. Positive reviews will certainly help the online reputation of the physician, potentially increasing the number of patients who will contact the office to set up an appointment. Negative reviews will most likely encourage the prospective patient to look for a different provider. To facilitate this process, many of these physician rating sites even suggest several physicians in that specialty located geographically nearby with higher ratings for the prospective patient.

What can be done by the provider who has a significant blemish on one or many of these physician rating sites? Unfortunately, the options on the physician rating site are rather limited. Most of the physician rating sites will not take down negative reviews, even if providers offer to pay. To do so would threaten the integrity of the Web site as a platform for opinions, both good and bad. However, many sites have a policy regarding what type of comments they will permit. For example, Healthgrades.com has a community review policy that states to respect others by not posting content that is harassing or uses profanity.[5] Some rating sites may offer "premium accounts," which has added features that put negative reviews lower in the profile by promoting more positive content.

These accounts are based on a subscription model. Besides providing higher search result placement, they offer additional tools that help diminish the impact of the negative review. For example, Healthgrades Advanced is $65 per month and Healthgrades Premium is $780 per month. Healthgrades Advanced removes advertisements as well as ads for competing providers. Healthgrades Premium adds patient testimonials and enhanced videos and photographs to better market the profile. The Healthgrades Premium account also provides the ability to promote the practice profile on competing physician profile pages as well as to be featured on the Healthgrades Web site. Therefore, despite a negative review, there are ways on many of these physician rating sites to promote your practice in the face of adversity.

Another potential strategy to fight negative reviews is to hire a lawyer and sue the patient, which a New York gynecologist did when a patient posted negative reviews on Yelp.[6] The patient posted negative reviews on Healthgrades.com and RateMDs. com as well to protest the "scare tactic" of blood tests and procedures to force her to book a second checkup appointment. Although the patient took down the negative online reviews, the lawsuit remained because the doctor stated that he suffered defamation, libel, and emotional stress from her comments stating that he was a "crook" and "scam artist." On 1 hand, hiring a lawyer and filing a lawsuit appears to be an appropriate way to defend one's reputation; however, in the context of mental health, some prospective patients may consider this action to be rather aggressive and not empathetic, steering them to consider alternate providers.

In lieu of hiring a lawyer, hiring a professional reputation firm, such as Reputation Defender[7] or WebiMax,[8] may be a better strategy. First, they conduct a discovery process of what information online is available and how that content impacts one's reputation. They then analyze the relative difficulty of removing or suppressing the negative content. One strategy to suppress negative content is to use search engine optimization so that more positive content bubbles up higher in search results and negative content moves to the back. The companies accomplish this strategy by creating new content and Web sites using metadata and link content on these pages to optimize search placement. These reputation services come at a cost of $3000 to $25,000 per year depending on the number of personalized Web sites, professional content, and unique direct Web sites desired.

A less expensive solution is that physicians should "claim" their profile on the rating sites. Although it may appear to be a Stockholm syndrome–type experience, claiming a physician rating profile and correcting erroneous information about the practice may positively impact how patients perceive your practice. In addition, a more accurate physician rating site will be found higher on search engine hits. It appears counterintuitive to help a site with negative reviews appear higher in search engine findings, but overall it is better exposure for your practice online. On that note, there are more than a dozen physician rating sites available. Although it is impossible to claim a profile on every site, consider at least every site listed on Kaitlyn Houseman's blog.[9]

Medical Practice Builders, a medical marketing firm, offers sound advice regarding how to respond to negative patient reviews.[10] They say that more than 90% of patient complaints are a result of miscommunication, which leads to patient dissatisfaction. It is key to not take complaints personally and do not become defensive or mad. Change the framework, and see a negative review as an opportunity to review and improve the patient experience. Respond to the patient in private and via a telephone call, which helps acknowledge their concerns and reengages the patient. It is much easier in conversation to identify tone and provide empathy and redirection than with words. Do not respond to reviews online because a response may lead to a HIPAA privacy breach because of the public nature of such communications. In addition, the temptation is too great when responding quickly online to write something that may be regretted later.

Another idea is to ask patients, friends, or staff to post positive reviews to drown out the negative ones. Although this strategy appears appropriate at first, it is risky because asking patients for reviews may be crossing a boundary in the psychiatrist-patient relationship. Having friends and staff post reviews is not a good idea because it is disingenuous and may be on that slippery slope of being unethical.

A better strategy to get more reviews is to have a card or sign in the office waiting room with a link to a physician review site for any review, not just positive ones. Likewise, office staff should not prompt or remind patients to review the practice, which will appear to be coercion, desperation, or both.

As mentioned previously by the medical marketing firm, the sting of negative reviews online hurts both professionally and personally. These reviews will evoke feelings such as disbelief, betrayal, and anger.

It is understandable that providers may become depressed and begin to experience self-doubt. However, they must recognize that the Internet has become the megaphone of dissent and bullying. Many providers have attended presentations where these issues are discussed at local and national meetings, and it is helpful to commiserate that one is not alone in this experience. Talking about one's experience to local trusted colleagues is also advised, as long as they will not judge and can provide support and advice. It is important to stay positive and maintain a balanced perspective, understanding fully that the many patients who are satisfied with their experience have not voiced these positive thoughts on the physician rating sites.

YOUR PRIVACY ONLINE

In the discovery process of determining what content online provides the grist for the mill of online reputation, providers will uncover more personal content that they wish would remain more private. Scott McNealy, former CEO of Sun Microsystems, is often quoted stating, "You have zero privacy anyway. Get over it."[11] However, despite this apparent truth, people still lock the door of their homes and secure their belongings instead of leaving doors unlocked or wide open. Unless someone has truly been always "off the grid" and no one has ever searched for information about that person, everyone has a digital footprint somewhere online.

The first step to mitigating privacy risks is to discover what information is out there. Keep in mind that some content may have been posted by other people and that one's identity has been "tagged." Search engines are the best tool for crawling the World Wide Web of content. When someone searches for information about a provider, creating an alert will notify that person.[12] Although the alert will not necessarily identify who is searching for a provider, it will provide at least some indication that someone is searching for information about that person and other terms of interest, such as "John, Luo, MD, psychiatry."[13]

Search engines are collecting information about everyone. Although it is impossible for it to erase everything that this company is collecting, Google does allow users some control over how much information it is collecting and when.[14] The Google Privacy Checkup tool works for those who have a Google account, namely its Gmail service. It allows users to pause location services, which tracks where one has been and what a user might need, such as directions to the next appointment. More importantly, it allows users to turn off what has been searched for and viewed on YouTube, akin to clearing cookies from a Web browser. Turning ad personalization off prevents Google from tracking items viewed and delivering specific ads. Although this level of granular detail is unlikely to be available to a prospective patient, at the same time, users may not even Google to have this level of detailed knowledge. One caveat is that some services may be useful to users, such as prediction of travel time to the next appointment, so there is a balancing act between user privacy and usability.

The adage that a picture is worth a thousand words is very true with regards to privacy. Health care providers should use Google Image search to see what pictures online have been linked to their name. It is often uncanny how accurate the search results are, and it is hoped that there are no photographs that are potentially compromising to one's reputation. Although Google only can track your online search activity and cannot delete photographs found on Web sites, knowing what can be seen by prospective patients and others is vital information. Google Image search is not the most comprehensive search for images, so checking popular photograph services, such as Photobucket.com, SmugMug.com, and Flickr.com, may reveal photographs tagged and linked to one's name uploaded by others. In addition, reverse image search, such as using TinEye.com, may also reveal what other sites may be hosting that same image. A photograph can be uploaded to TinEye.com or on a Web page; right-click over a photograph to copy the image address and paste it into reverse search engine. This service may be useful to discover if an image has "gone viral" and has been copied for use on other sites on the Internet.

Shopping sites, such as Amazon.com, have dominated with the features and services it has to offer. Wish lists, such as Giftster.com, help decrease the need to return gifts in addition to helping gift givers figure out what to purchase. However, those profiles online can contain information, such as hometown or a birth date, that can be used to further help identify users on other Web sites. Adjust the privacy settings on these accounts so that a list is shared only with friends and family and not publicly viewable or searchable by search engines. It may be necessary to send an e-mail to these people to access the list, and although that may take some effort, it will improve your privacy in the long run.

In this era of "big data" with online activity being tracked and user profiles collected online, there are simple and effective steps to fight for one's privacy. First, do not sign into a Google account, such as Gmail. All Web browsing will be tracked and linked to this account unless one has adjusted the privacy setting as described earlier. Even if one has not signed into a Gmail account, Google is tracking all Web searches based on the IP address of the computer. Fortunately, multiple users on a network, such as a wireless access point, have an internal IP address, so the search information and site visitation of all users will be aggregated together, and individual profiles will be difficult to determine.

Adding an extension or browser plug-in to a Web browser is one way to add additional security to protect privacy. For example, the popular Chrome Web browser has a myriad of third-party developed extensions to improve security. Privacy Badger, a product of the Electronic Frontier Foundation (EFF; Eff.org), helps block invisible trackers and spying ads. Another useful extension from the EFF is HTTPS Everywhere, which encrypts communication with major Web sites, thereby making browsing more secure. Noiszy is a browser plug-in that creates meaningless Web browsing data. In summary, it hits all trackers and crawlers on a Web site to pollute your data stream, which will confound algorithms collecting data about you and burst the filter bubble that specifies what searches are directed higher for you. One caveat about installing too many browser extensions is that they do take up computer CPU cycles, which may impact your computer speed and productivity. It may be easier to use DuckDuckGo.com or StartPage.com as the default Web page, which are homepage sites that provide more private searching. They do not store any information about browsing history nor do they bubble up products or sites based on clicks or sites visited. Qwant.com is a European-based Chrome browser search engine extension that also does not collect personal information and guarantees neutrality and impartiality of search results. Last, there are secure browsers, such as Epic or Brave, which are based on the Chrome browser source code but hardened to block ads and trackers. To test the ability of these tools to block trackers, the EFF has created Panopticlick, a Web site that will run tests to see how good a job the browser blocks nonconsensual Web tracking.[15]

Social media sites, such as Facebook.com, may potentially reveal personal information unless the right security settings are set. Twitter.com tweets may reveal interesting information about providers and his or her opinions depending on whether posts are personal or professional in nature. Management of privacy on these sites requires spending the time to adjust the settings to allow only friends to see posts or to require approval of followers. Apple iPhone users are in luck that an app, Jumbo (https://www.jumboprivacy.com/), will take care of managing privacy on Facebook, Twitter, Google search, and Alexa with Instagram and Tinder in development. Once installed on the iPhone, it asks for users to log in on each of these sites, which is stored locally on the phone and not linked to a user account. Running the app periodically will then scrub online activity with a simple touch on the "start cleaning" button.

Although it may be alarming what general information that search engines such as Google collect, people search sites, such as Pipl.com, Spokeo.com, and TruePeopleSearch.com, may reveal more personal and therefore frightening information. These sites search social media, public records, real estate property records, telephone numbers, addresses, and more. For example, using city information from an Amazon profile, a search for a common name, such as "John Smith," will help further reduce the number of potential matches. The profile information includes current address, previous addresses, telephone numbers, associated names of relatives, and names of other potential associates. The results are frightening because of the accuracy of the information. In patient care, these sites may be useful in finding relatives for patients who have wandered away from their homes, but for providers, this information may impact the therapeutic relationship. Fortunately, many of these sites do offer record removal requests for privacy purposes. Information online, such as the Surveillance Self-Defense (https://ssd.eff.org/) from the EFF and RestorePrivacy. com, provides a summary of tools to help providers combat the invasion of privacy.

PROFESSIONAL USE OF SOCIAL MEDIA

When social media sites, such as Facebook and LinkedIn, started more than a dozen years ago, there was a distinct separation between personal and professional social media use. Facebook started at first by only allowing students, faculty, and staff to create accounts. Their number of users skyrocketed when they allowed anyone to create an account and added more tools and applications, such as games. LinkedIn was by invitation only in the beginning, but soon opened its doors to anyone to create an account.

In recent years, the boundaries between professional and personal use of social media sites began to blur. Facebook actively promotes business use on their site, and LinkedIn added many features, such as likes and newsfeeds, to become more personal in nature.

Over the years, professional use of social media has been transformed. At first, there was practically a strict adherence to avoid any use of social media professionally to avoid HIPAA violations, and for psychiatrists, potential boundary crossings with patients by revealing too much personal information. Medical schools had educational sessions about social media use and how that personal information may potentially have an impact on their future careers. Indeed, resident physicians on recruitment committees could look up a medical student's Facebook account and see content there that lowered the student's position on the program rank order list. A YouTube video of an intoxicated and agitated neurology resident ultimately led to her dismissal in the last year of her residency program.[16] Now, many health care providers and organizations have embraced social media use in professional practice.

The key to professional use of social media is exactly that, keeping it professional. There are a growing number of Facebook accounts for medical and psychiatric practices. It makes sense because these social media sites have such stickiness, and the public is increasingly using these sites as their "homepage." Having a practice presence on Facebook may lower the barrier for patients to consider seeing a psychiatrist. Twitter has been typically used for marketing but now has a role in extending and establishing a brand for individuals, organizations, and health care facilities. The MedEdChat (https://twitter.com/MedEdChat) hosts a forum on Twitter on Thursdays at 9 PM Eastern time. Even YouTube and Instagram have provided opportunities for hospitals and organizations to showcase their educational and professional services, awards, and humanitarian efforts.

To guide the health care provider, in the code of ethics, the American Medical Association has a policy on professional use of social media.[17] This code includes language commenting on patient privacy and confidentiality, informed consent, and boundary issues. The American Psychiatric Association has a guide on the use of social media for psychiatrists.[18] This toolkit covers LinkedIn, Facebook, Twitter, and Instagram and how to use these tools to educate patients and fight the stigma of mental illness. The Mayo Clinic has created a social media network that offers a conference, blog-based information, Webinars, and even a 1-day "residency" regarding social media use.[19] With all these resources and gradual adjustment of attitudes, social media in health care will certainly continue to evolve and expand.

Table 1
Top 10 recommendations for maintaining privacy online and improving your online reputation

Recommendation	Example Action
1. Search for information about yourself online	Search for your name on Google.com, Bing.com, or Search.Yahoo.com and review findings
2. Check for ratings on physician rating sites	Search for your name on Vitals.com, Healthgrades.com, and RateMDs.com
3. Claim your provider profile on physician rating sites	Take ownership of information on physician rating sites, update any invalid content, and periodically monitor for any ratings and comments
4. Respond to negative reviews on physician rating sites if patient is identifiable	Respond in person or over the telephone, not on the physician rating site. Do not be defensive, listen empathetically, and provide a corrective action if possible
5. Invite all patients to review your practice on various physician rating sites	Create business cards with links to various physician ratings sites on the back; if URL length is a concern, truncate the URL using TinyURL.com
6. Create search alerts to identify when someone is searching for you and what they may be reviewing	Create alerts on Google.com/alerts, Talkwaker.com/alerts, and Anewstip.com/alerts
7. Update privacy settings on various sites with personal information	Revise profile on Amazon.com, change settings on FaceBook.com and Google Privacy Checkup
8. Check image searches to see what has been posted	Use Images.Google.com and search your name on popular sites, such as PhotoBucket.com, SmugMug.com, and Flickr.com
9. Harden your privacy online by blocking Web trackers and spying ads	Add browser plug-ins, such as Privacy Badger, BlockSite, AdGuard Adblocker, and uBlock Origin or use a secure browser such as Epic or Brave
10. Check for personal information using people search engines and request removal	Search for yourself on Pipl.com, Spokeo.com, and TruePeopleSearch.com and remove your profile

SUMMARY

This article has provided an overview of how the Internet and the information contained therein has had an impact on reputation and privacy for health care providers. The amount of content online is vastly overwhelming, and it may be impossible to ascertain all the content available that plays a role in how prospective patients perceive us. Potential damage to one's online reputation is much too easily accomplished with the advent of physician rating and social media sites. Privacy in all practicality does not exist online, and artificial intelligence and other tools are poised to make discovering information on the psychiatrist Dr John Smith all that much easier to find. The information on the Internet clearly has both positive and negative uses, and although there are almost too many tools out there to use to improve privacy yet maintain communication, learning about some of them is a must for today's practitioner (**Table 1**). It is important to be resilient, educated, and mindful that it is a new climate to which we must adapt on a daily basis.

REFERENCES

1. Strickland J. How ARPANET works. Available at: https://computer.howstuffworks. com/arpanet.htm. Accessed February 23, 2019.
2. Bosman J. After 244 years, Encyclopaedia Britannica stops the presses. Available at: https://mediadecoder.blogs.nytimes.com/2012/03/13/after-244-years-encyclopaedia-britannica-stops-the-presses/. Accessed February 23, 2019.
3. American Medical Association Doctor Finder. Available at: https://doctorfinder. ama-assn.org/doctorfinder/home.jsp. Accessed February 24, 2019.
4. Howley EK. How to find the best primary care doctor. Available at: https://health. usnews.com/health-care/patient-advice/articles/2018-01-09/how-to-find-the-best-primary-care-doctor. Accessed February 24, 2019.
5. Healthgrades community review guidelines. Available at: https://www. healthgrades.com/content/community-review-guidelines. Accessed April 2, 2019.
6. Fearnow B. NYC gynecologist files $1 million lawsuit over negative yelp reviews 2018. Available at: https://www.newsweek.com/joon-song-bad-review-yelp-lawsuit-gynecologist-michelle-levine-defamation-new-950538. Accessed April 30, 2019.
7. Reputation defender. Available at: https://www.reputationdefender.com/lp/business/. Accessed April 2, 2019.
8. WebiMax. Available at: https://webimax.com. Accessed April 30, 2019.
9. Houseman K. 10 most popular physician rating and review sites. Available at: https://www.grouponehealthsource.com/blog/10-most-popular-physician-rating-and-review-sites. Accessed April 30, 2019.
10. How to respond to negative patient reviews online. Available at: https://www. medpb.com/how-to-respond-to-negative-patient-reviews-online/. Accessed April 30, 2019.
11. Noyes K. Scott McNealy on privacy: you still don't have any. Available at: https:// www.pcworld.com/article/2941052/scott-mcnealy-on-privacy-you-still-dont-have-any.html. Accessed May 1, 2019.
12. Google search alert. Available at: https://support.google.com/websearch/answer/4815696?hl=en. Accessed April 13, 2019.
13. Knapp J. How to set up a Google Alert (and why it is a good idea). Available at: https://www.bloggingbasics101.com/how-to-set-up-a-google-alert-and-why-its-a-good-idea/. Accessed May 1, 2019.

14. Haselton T. Google collects information about many things you do online–here is how to stop it. Available at: https://www.cnbc.com/2019/05/01/how-to-stop-google-from-collecting-your-private-information.html. Accessed May 1, 2019.
15. Panopticlick. Available at: https://panopticlick.eff.org/. Accessed May 1, 2019.
16. Doctor accused of attacking Uber driver: 'I'm Ashamed' | ABC News. Available at: https://www.youtube.com/watch?v=kExGmpGTdl0. Accessed May 1, 2019.
17. AMA. Professionalism in the use of social media. Available at: https://www.ama-assn.org/delivering-care/ethics/professionalism-use-social-media. Accessed May 1, 2019.
18. APA best practices for social media. Available at: https://www.psychiatry.org/psychiatrists/practice/social-media. Accessed May 1, 2019.
19. Mayo Clinic Social Media Network. Available at: https://socialmedia.mayoclinic.org/. Accessed May 1, 2019.

Intended and Unintended Consequence in the Digital Age of Psychiatry

The Interface of Culture and Technology in Psychiatric Treatments

Jay H. Shore, MD, MPH

KEYWORDS

- Technology • Cultural • Mental health • Telepsychiatry • Telemental health
- e-mental health

KEY POINTS

- As providers and health care systems navigate the evolving health care landscape, they should take steps to account for the impact of the technology culture interface on clinical processes.
- Individual providers should consider including as part of their initial intake a cultural assessment that includes not only appropriate elements related to cultural issues but also patients' past experience and perspectives on technologies.
- Providers should be aware of their own experiences and perspectives on technologies and how these may influence their interactions with patients including biases and limitations inherent in the technologies they are using.
- Health care systems should pay attention to the technology culture interfaces as they develop, adapt, and deploy technologies in clinical settings. This includes monitoring impact on both the shaping of clinical content as well as process.
- As a field, psychiatry needs to develop frameworks for formally evaluating the use of existing and innovating technologies for use in mental health treatment.

INTRODUCTION

Psychiatry is experiencing a period of unprecedented evolution driven by larger societal forces. The latter part of the twentieth century saw the transition of society from an

---

Disclosure: Dr J.H. Shore is the Chief Medical Officer of AccessCare, a company that provides telebehavioral health services.
Department of Psychiatry and Family Medicine, School of Medicine, Centers for American Indian and Alaska Native Health, Colorado School of Public Health, Telemedicine Helen and Arthur E. Johnson Depression Center, University of Colorado Anschutz Medical Campus, 13055 East 17th, Avenue, F800, Aurora, CO 80045, USA
E-mail address: jay.shore@ucdenver.edu

Psychiatr Clin N Am 42 (2019) 659–668
https://doi.org/10.1016/j.psc.2019.08.008
0193-953X/19/© 2019 Elsevier Inc. All rights reserved.

industrial to technology base ushering changes in societal organization and function. This ongoing transition is transforming research, organization, and care delivery systems within Western Medicine including psychiatry. Because psychiatry, especially in the United States, is undergoing technological transformation; it is also facing fundamental alterations to its structure driven by funding challenges that are continuously shaped by changing treatments, demographics, and political vicissitudes.

Culture plays a critical role in shaping the structure, content, and process of medical and psychiatric treatment. Although historically underappreciated, in recent decades there has been a growing acknowledgment of the impact of culture on medicine. Increasingly, there is also a recognition of the influence of culture on the development, implementation, and use of technology. This influence experienced in society in general is also affecting medical and mental health care. The culture and technology interface has significant potential to affect clinical processes and outcomes. Despite the widespread and expanding deployment of technology in psychiatry there is a paucity of information of the effect of the technology and cultural interactions on clinical work.

The purpose of this article is to review the impact of the cultural and technology interface on psychiatric care and to proffer a pragmatic approach to examine and appreciate this influence. The article begins with a review of how historical forces have shaped the development of medicine, technology, and mental health and how these converge in the delivery of current clinical care. A framework is presented to help psychiatric providers understand the interplay of cultural and technology on patient-provider interactions and dynamics. The article concludes with strategies for individual providers and mental health care systems to address the culture technology interface.

HISTORICAL CONVERGENCE OF MEDICINE, TECHNOLOGY, AND MENTAL HEALTH

A recent review of the evolution and history of telepsychiatry in *International Review of Psychiatry* presents a narrative on the development of our current industrialized system of medicine.[1] Systems of medicine arise from the culture of the societies in which they are embedded. Agrarian and Indigenous tribal societies create forms of community-based medicine with care occurring at a patient's location. The trajectory of Western Medicine shaped in concert with the growth of Western Civilization is one of centralization followed by industrialization. The early medical schools of the Greeks and Persians began the trend of consolidation of medical learning to centers of excellence in population dense areas.[2] This trend was further reinforced in the middles ages by the urbanization of hospitals growing from the hospice system.[3] Current health care is dominated by urbanized academic and nonacademic hospitals systems that continue to consolidate, merge, and centralize control and access to medical treatment. As western society shifted to industrial means of production, Western Medicine adopted an industrial model of care, which reached its pinnacle in the last 50 years.[4] This is illustrated in the organization of health care systems using production line models and the commodification of medicine.[5]

In reaction to this model there have been attempts to reconceptualize the funding of health care (product vs right, private vs public) as well as attempts to redirect its focus. The seminal Institute of Medicine, *Crossing the Quality Chasm,* called for more personalized, patient-center care, closer to the patient with improvements in quality and cost.[6] This calls for increased focused on quality and cost in health care contributed to the often publicly lauded "Triple and Quadruple Aims" framework, improving population health and patient experience while reducing costs and provider burnout, a benchmark guide for many in health care policy.[7] Challenges within the industrial medical model and attempts to reform the model have played out recently, at least in the

United States, during a time of incredible dynamism, change, and uncertainty for health care funding. Psychiatry and mental health care in the form of integrated care has been put forth as important component for decreasing overall costs and improving quality and outcomes in medical care.[8] Efforts to enhance or shift models of funding and care have been enabled through the increasing use of technology in medicine.

The end of the twentieth century heralded a tectonic shift in western civilization from an industrial to information age. Exponential acceleration of microprocessors in the 1970s enabled the rise of personal computing, Internet, and mobile technologies in the 1980s and 1990s, driving fundamental shifts in the organization and means of production in society. Technology has been put forth as a key enabler in medicine and psychiatry to help shift models to more patient centric and higher-quality care while decreasing costs.[1] Although medicine and psychiatry have been quick to adapt and implement certain technologies, this adaptation has arguably been used to reenforce industrial structures and systems of care rather than to truly shift from an industrial to information age model due to both the design process for medical technology as well as the underlying funding structures that support and reenforce a more traditional industrial medical model. Dr Peter Yellowlees puts forth, called here "Yellowlees's Corollary":

> Computers never forget and are excellent at scheduling, reminding, and remembering, but humans are still much, much better at data analysis and decision making....We need to make sure that we use computers ....for what they are best at, and that we do not forget or set aside the honed human skills in pattern recognition and data interpretation that are essential to the diagnostic process and that make psychiatrists such sensitive and broadly trained physicians....it is essential to redesign business processes before introducing or developing new software environments.[9]

A classic example of unintended consequences of technology design and implementation is the modern electronic medical record (EMR). Purportedly introduced into the health care system to improve quality of care through improved patient documentation, decreased medical error, and improved medical communication, much of its design has been focused on improving encounter tracking and coding to maximize reimbursement. Physician and patient are troubled with the EHR interference on clinical interactions and its contribution to the acceleration of physician burnout.[10,11] A study of emergency department physicians demonstrated they spend most of their time in charting (43%) as compared with direct patient care (28%), averaging more than 4000 mouse clicks per 10 hour shift.[12]

In The authors revisit unintended consequences in the deployment of technology in psychiatry and delve deeper into the additional impact that cultural has in later discussion. Key concepts of technology in psychiatry as well as the role of cultural in mental health are discussed in the following section.

TECHNOLOGY IN PSYCHIATRY

Two relatively recent emerging rubrics of the interface of technology in psychiatry are relevant for this discussion. The first rubric defines the extent of which a technology is used in everyday psychiatric practice. The term "base technologies" has been used to refer to those technologies that have already been adapted; are in wide spread daily use; have a body of evidence and experience supporting their deployment; and consist of email, the Internet, mobile devices (including the telephone), live interactive videoconferencing, and the EMR. *Emergent* technologies are those that have more limited or pilot use, less accumulated evidence on their value, have not been widely diffused, and face unclear future as to their widespread adoption. Examples include virtual reality, virtual worlds, voice and face recognition, and positional tracking.[13]

The second rubric is a more widely held conceptualization, dating back to 2001, that explains our changing society and has important current implications for the psychiatry and technology interface, "digital natives" versus "digital immigrants." Digital natives are defined as the generation that was born into and came of age with our modern technologies and are assumed to be more comfortable with technology, more tech savvy, have greater access to technology, and more at ease with the pace of technological change. Digital immigrants are people who did not grow up with technology and began being exposed and learning technology in their adult life. Digital immigrants are thought to be more wary of technology, use it less, and take longer to adapt and ingrate it.[14] This lexicon has gained traction in many spheres, with a review by Wang and colleagues[15] proposing a more nuanced view drawing attention to recent literature showing a less discreet generational divide and more of a continuum versus bimodal conceptualization of attitudes toward technology. They propose the concept of "digital fluency," defining it as the ability to not only knowing how to use technology but also to leverage to produce "things of significance." The authors go on to proffer a 7-factor model that shapes digital fluency: demographic characteristics, psychological factors, social influences, educational factors, behavioral intention, opportunity, and actual use of technology.[15] These factors can be leveraged in understanding an individual patient or psychiatrist's past exposure to technology, their digital fluency and where they land, and the digital immigrant-digital native continuum. The factors are part of the overall patient and provider cultural backgrounds that affect clinical processes and the psychiatrist/patient relationship.

ROLE OF CULTURE IN MENTAL HEALTH

The importance of the impact of culture in medicine and psychiatry is critical and ubiquitous. There is a plethora of definitions of culture in the anthropological literature. A broad and classic definition taken from Spradley and McCurdy, "The acquired knowledge that people use to interpret their world and generate social behavior is called culture. Culture is not behavior itself."[16] The medical literature in general and behavioral literature specifically is replete with examples of the impact of culture on clinical care, including its impact on patient-provider rapport, treatment engagement, and clinical outcomes.[17–20]

The importance of addressing culture in medical treatments has been codified in the move toward cultural competence defined ambitiously for mental health by the US Surgeon General in 2001 as

The delivery of mental health services that are responsive to the cultural and linguistic concerns of all racial or ethnic minority and non-minority group, including their psychosocial issues, characteristic styles of problem presentation, family, and immigration histories traditions, beliefs and values.[17]

Cultural competence has increased attention to cultural issues not only in clinical care but within health care organizations themselves. Cultural competence has been further refined by the idea "cultural humility," which envisions culture competency as a process rather than an end product.[21] Cultural humility challenges the idea that a provider can truly become completely cultural fluent in another culture and challenges one to remain open and aware of the limitations of knowledge of other cultures through 3 fundamental tenants for providers: (1) a life-long commitment to self-evaluation and critique; (2) desire to collaborate with patient to address power imbalance in shared cultural knowledge in the provider-patient relationships; and (3) interest to work with others to address power imbalance due to culture at the systems level. The stances of both culture competence and culture humility strive toward Substance Abuse and Mental health Services Administration's more succinct definition of cultural competence, "The ability to interact effectively with people of different cultures."[22]

Psychiatry has led other fields in medicine in acknowledging, framing, and addressing cultural issues in clinical care. The Diagnostic and Statistical Manual (DSM) recommends a framework for addressing culture in clinical treatment through the cultural formulation, which directs psychiatrist to examine 4 important components in a clinical interaction: (1) the cultural identity of the patient; (2) a patient's cultural conceptualization of distress; (3) the patient's psychosocial stressors and cultural features of vulnerability and resilience; and (4) how cultural features of the relationship between the individual and the clinician affect the clinical interactions. The psychiatrist after accounting for these factors then creates an overall cultural assessment intended to summarize the relevant cultural components and their implications for diagnosis and appropriate management and interventions. Originally created for DSM-IV, DSM-V further refined the cultural formulation as well as suggested the cultural formulation interview, a set of 16 questions for clinicians to use as appropriate to more systematically assess the impact of culture on key aspects of a patient's clinical presentation.[23]

Although acknowledged at times as a peripheral factor, culture at the interface of technology and psychiatry has rarely been addressed as a main thematic topic. The bulk of the mental health technology and culture literature has come from telepsychiatry, live interactive videoconferencing, with the major focus being the feasibility of conducting and adapting videoconferencing to increase access to underserved minority populations. Only a handful of articles have explored the impact of technology and culture on clinical process. And only one has specifically focused on this, entitled "Cultural Aspects of Telepsychiatry." In this article, the authors address each area of the DSM-IV Cultural Formulation highlighting components that are particularly relevant to telepsychiatry. One important component is how the cultural background of patients influences their comfort and attitude toward telepsychiatry. Another one is how telepsychiatry can emphasize patient and provider differences created by differing locations, such as difference between rural and urban culture.[24] This latter issue is relevant to all technologies in use in psychiatry. Both base and emergent technologies in psychiatry create the ability to instantaneously transmute distance and time, allowing psychiatrist and patient to communicate without awareness of the cultural and environmental contexts in which each is situated. This issue is acknowledged in the article around telepsychiatry, with the authors recommending psychiatrist pursue several solutions to increase awareness and familiarity across the patient and provider settings.[24]

Although this article began to examine these important factors, there has been a dearth in the literature of exploring these issues further or the occurrence of these issues in other technologies being deployed in psychiatry. More importantly, the critical issue of the impact of cultural and cultural bias on the development, adaptation, and use of technology in society and medicine has not been addressed. This unseen influence may have wide current and future impact on psychiatrist-patient relationships, processes, and outcomes.

CULTURAL INFLUENCES ON TECHNOLOGY DEVELOPMENT

The end user of a technology is unaware of the design work, processes, and assumptions that created the end product for their use. Technology in our society is driven and created by the dominant culture, the influence of which is only just now being more widely examined for society and has yet to be scrutinized in detail in medicine or psychiatry. Important illustrations of these biases involve search engine biases driven by their design and core algorithms. It was recently revealed how search engine algorithms in Google delivered stereotypical imagines of African American youth compared with Caucasian reinforced through the biases of searches conducted by members of the dominant society.[25] Even more concerning is a recent report by the Georgetown Law's Center on Privacy and Technology on the use of facial recognition technology by law enforcement. This report catalogs how biases and inaccuracies in the core programming, algorithms, inherent user/system biases, and training and deployment of these systems disproportionately affect minority communities.[26]

A large randomized controlled study demonstrated how biased search engine rankings can shift voter preference by more than 20%, targeting specific demographic groups and be masked from the targeted groups, labeled the "manipulation effect" by the investigators.[27] Another controlled study demonstrated how manipulating search engine selection and sorting criteria could affect users seeking health information on vaccination belief and attitudes. The study showed that biased results could change users' opinions independent of users' assessment of site credibility, suggesting users were unaware of the factors steering them to credible versus biases sources of information.[28] Closer to home, a randomized online study looked at confirmation bias in web-based search evaluation of expert information and social tags on the public evaluating information around the effectiveness of pharmacology versus psychotherapy for the treatment of depression. This study concluded that social tags/links to blog could heavily influence user opinion about which treatments are most effective bringing opinion closer in line with the scientific evidence.[29]

The body of literature in this area shows that not only does the development and programming of technology create risk of biases but user adaptation creates additional risks and opportunities for miscommunication in medical technologies. This becomes especially salient as our systems of care increases its adaptation of technologies in many, whose use behind the scenes, such as the EMR or population registries, has yet to be examined for biases that affect clinical decision-making and treatment. In addition, the increased volume of information being generated by medical technology systems, as in the previous example of EMRs in the emergency department, also create challenges for provider information overload as psychiatrist try and sort through signal to noise issues for information in patients for which they provide care. Although artificial intelligence (AI) is being proposed as a solution to support physicians to manage this growing data, significant concerns have been raised by inherent biases in AI's core programming. Of even greater concern is that the growing complexity of AI systems has made it extremely challenging to determine and track the internal processes by which AI reach their fundamental conclusions.[30]

CULTURE AND TECHNOLOGY IN PSYCHIATRY

Proffered in **Fig. 1** is a framework intended to aid psychiatric providers in attending to the interplay and impact of cultural and technology on patient-provider interactions, processes, and dynamics.

This framework is presented to help psychiatric providers develop and understand the interplay of cultural and technology on patient-provider interactions and dynamics.

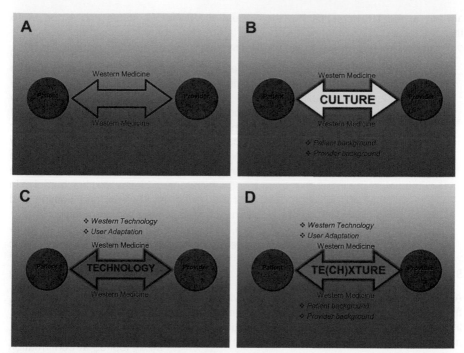

Fig. 1. (*A–D*) Cultural framework for assessing impact of interplay of cultural and technology on patient-provider interactions.

Fig. 1A presents Western Medicine as the baseline framework/boundaries in which the provider-patient interaction occurs.

Fig. 1B demonstrates the overlay of cultural on the provider-patient interaction within the context of western medicine with attention to key areas, along the lines of DSM-V formulation, that influence these interactions including patient background issues (cultural identity of the individual, cultural concepts of distress, environmental factors) and provider background issues (cultural features affecting the interactions). Additional attention is also needed around the provider's and patient's past experiences with technology including exposure (digital immigrant vs digital native) and digital fluency.

Fig. 1C shows overlay of technology on the provider-patient interaction within in the context of western medicine. Two key issues in this area are the impact of technologies underlying structure, programming, and assumptions on the communication process as well as how user adaptation further alters the technologies' influence on clinical process.

Fig. 1D shows the complete framework, combining **Fig. 1**A–C, for consideration and using the work "techture" to represent and draw attention to the combination of culture and technology influences on clinical processes within the context of Western medicine.

What follows is an illustrative case example of how this framework can be applied: a 55-year-old white male psychiatrist working with a 19-year-old Hispanic woman whose parents are immigrants from Bolivia. She is being treated for depression with medication and a course of cognitive behavioral therapy. They are communicating between sessions through texting (using an HIPPA secure texting platform) initially around scheduling logistics but then about the patient's status and mood state through texting abbreviations and emojis. In monitoring the impact of this discourse on the provider-patient relationships the psychiatrist should consider the following:

- How their background exposure and experience with technology in general and texting specifically may influence their communication (digital immigrant vs digital native, digital fluency).
- How the technologies' medium for communication (abbreviations and symbols) influences the following: what is communicated by each and how that communication is interpreted and meaning is constructed.
- How their different cultural backgrounds (gender, ethnicity, age, education) may add additional contributions to interpretation by each to the bidirectional communication.
- The psychiatrist should be mindful of the possibility of miscommunication and have a low threshold to seek additional clarification around meaning through a different form of communication (eg, in-person session or by phone if more urgent, should a safety issue or concern arise).

SUMMARY

As providers and health care systems navigate the evolving health care landscape, they should take steps to account for the impact of "techture" on clinical processes. Individual providers should consider including as part of their initial intake a cultural assessment that includes not only appropriate elements related to cultural issues but also patients' past experience and perspectives on technologies. Providers should be aware of their own experiences and perspectives on technologies and how these may influence their interactions with patients including biases and limitations inherent in the technologies they are using. Psychiatrist should monitor in an ongoing fashion the impact of "techture" on clinical processes including comfort, rapport, and communication.

Health care systems should pay attention to "techture" as they develop, adapt, and deploy technologies in clinical settings. This includes monitoring impact on both the shaping of clinical content as well as process. As a field, psychiatry needs to develop frameworks for formally evaluating the use of existing and innovating technologies for use in mental health treatment. This will require the conceptualization of new configurations of development and evaluation teams with a multidisplinary approach to include IT, engineering, social science, patients, and their communities as a multi-stage iterative and adaptive approach to better integrating technology into mental health care.

REFERENCES

1. Shore J. The evolution and history of telepsychiatry and its impact on psychiatric care: Current implications for psychiatrists and psychiatric organizations. Int Rev Psychiatry 2015;27(6):469-75.
2. Modanlou HD. Historical evidence for the origin of teaching hospital, medical school and the rise of academic medicine. J Perinatol 2011;31(4):236-9.
3. Riva MA, Cesana G. The charity and the care: the origin and the evolution of hospitals. Eur J Intern Med 2013;24(1):1-4.
4. Szreter S. Industrialization and health. Br Med Bull 2004;69(1):75-86.
5. Varkey P, Reller MK, Resar RK. Basics of quality improvement in health care. Mayo Clin Proc 2007;82(6):735-9.

6. Institute of Medicine (US) committee on quality of health care in America. Washington, DC: National Academies Press (US); 2001.
7. Bodenheimer T, Sinsky C. From triple to quadruple aim: care of the patient requires care of the provider. Ann Fam Med 2014;12(6):573–6.
8. Blount A, Schoenbaum M, Kathol R, et al. The economics of behavioral health services in medical settings: a summary of the evidence. Prof Psychol Res Pr 2007; 38(3):290.
9. Yellowlees P, Nafiz N. The psychiatrist-patient relationship of the future: anytime, anywhere? Harv Rev Psychiatry 2010;18(2):96–102.
10. Shachak A, Reis S. The impact of electronic medical records on patient–doctor communication during consultation: a narrative literature review. J Eval Clin Pract 2009;15(4):641–9.
11. Shanafelt TD, Dyrbye LN, Sinsky C, et al. Relationship between clerical burden and characteristics of the electronic environment with physician burnout and professional satisfaction. Mayo Clin Proc 2016;91(7):836–48.
12. Hill RG, Sears LM, Melanson SW. 4000 clicks: a productivity analysis of electronic medical records in a community hospital ED. Am J Emerg Med 2013;31(11): 1591–4.
13. Yellowless P, Shore J. Telepsychiatry and health technologies: a guide for mental health professionals. American Psychiatric Association Publishing; 2018.
14. Prensky M. Digital natives, digital immigrants part 1. Horizon 2001;9(5):1–6.
15. Wang QE, Myers MD, Sundaram D. Digital natives and digital immigrants-towards a model of digital fluency. Business & Information Systems Engineering 2013;5(6):409–19.
16. Spradley JP, McCurdy DW. Conformity and conflict: readings in cultural anthropology. Jill Potash; 2012.
17. United States. Public Health Service, Office of the Surgeon General, Center for Mental Health Services (US), United States, Substance Abuse, Mental Health Services Administration, National Institute of Mental Health (US). Mental health: culture, race, and ethnicity: a supplement to mental health: a report of the surgeon general. Department of Health and Human Services, US Public Health Service; 2001.
18. Corrigan PW, Druss BG, Perlick DA. The impact of mental illness stigma on seeking and participating in mental health care. Psychol Sci Public Interest 2014;15(2):37–70.
19. Betancourt JR, Green AR, Carrillo JE, et al. Defining cultural competence: a practical framework for addressing racial/ethnic disparities in health and health care. Public Health Rep 2016;118(4):293–302.
20. Truong M, Paradies Y, Priest N. Interventions to improve cultural competency in healthcare: a systematic review of reviews. BMC Health Serv Res 2014;14(1):99.
21. American Psychological Association. Available at: http://www.apa.org/pi/families/resources/newsletter/2013/08/cultural-humility.aspx. Accessed December 3, 2017.
22. Cultural Competence [Internet]. Cultural Competence | SAMHSA. Available at: http://www.samhsa.gov/capt/applying-strategic-prevention/cultural-competence. Accessed December 3, 2017.
23. American Psychiatric Association diagnostic and statistical manual of mental disorders. 5th edition. Arlington (VA): American Psychiatric Publishing; 2013. p. 5–25.
24. Shore JH, Savin DM, Novins D, et al. Cultural aspects of telepsychiatry. J Telemed Telecare 2006;12(3):116–21.

25. Guarino B. Google faulted for racial bias in image search results for black teen-agers. Washington (DC): WP Company; 2016. Available at: https://www.washingtonpost.com/news/morning-mix/wp/2016/06/10/google-faulted-for-racial-bias-in-image-search-results-for-black-teenagers. Accessed December 3, 2017.
26. Garvie C. The perpetual line-up: unregulated police face recognition in America. Washington (DC): Georgetown Law, Center on Privacy & Technology; 2016. Report dealing inherent biases in technology development and programming.
27. Epstein R, Robertson RE. The search engine manipulation effect (SEME) and its possible impact on the outcomes of elections. Proc Natl Acad Sci U S A 2015; 112(33):E4512–21.
28. Allam A, Schulz PJ, Nakamoto K. The impact of search engine selection and sort-ing criteria on vaccination beliefs and attitudes: two experiments manipulating Google output. J Med Internet Res 2014;16(4):e100.
29. Schweiger S, Oeberst A, Cress U. Confirmation bias in web-based search: a ran-domized online study on the effects of expert information and social tags on in-formation search and evaluation. J Med Internet Res 2014;16(3):e94.
30. Kuang C. Can A.I. Be Taught to explain itself? The New York Times 2017. Available at: https://www.nytimes.com/2017/11/21/magazine/can-ai-be-taught-to-explain-itself.html. Accessed December 3, 2017.

University of California Technology Wellness Index

A Physician-Centered Framework to Assess Technologies' Impact on Physician Well-Being

Keisuke Nakagawa, MD*, Peter M. Yellowlees, MBBS, MD

KEYWORDS

- Burnout • Technology • Health technology • Physician well-being • Physician health
- Electronic medical record • Wellness

KEY POINTS

- We have developed the University of California Technology Wellness Index (UCTWI), modeled on Stanford's WellMD Professional Fulfillment Index and the Institute for Healthcare Improvement's Quadruple Aim, to provide a fast, systematic, physician-centered framework to assess the impact of technologies on physician well-being.
- Many of the important factors that contribute to physician burnout are overlooked when introducing new technologies to clinical environments.
- Given that the pace of research is much slower than the rate of technological innovation, organizations often lack reliable methods to evaluate the potential impact of new technologies on physician health and well-being.
- To our knowledge, there is no tool available for health care organizations to quickly and systematically assess technology's impact on physician well-being. We demonstrate telepsychiatry use cases where the UCTWI is useful.
- Technologies like telepsychiatry have demonstrated positive effects on physician well-being by saving physicians time, enhancing work-life balance, improving quality, and restoring more control and flexibility to physicians' practices, whereas such technologies as electronic medical records (EMRs) have historically contributed to worsening physician burnout by reducing time with physicians and increasing time spent on documentation.

How many physicians would seriously consider going back to paper charts? Technologies, such as electronic medical records (EMRs), are often criticized for contributing to physician burnout.[1,2] EMRs have caused physicians to spend more time staring at

Disclosure Statement: The authors have nothing to disclose.
Department of Psychiatry and Behavioral Sciences, UC Davis Health, 2230 Stockton Boulevard, Sacramento, CA 95817, USA
* Corresponding author.
E-mail address: drknakagawa@ucdavis.edu

Psychiatr Clin N Am 42 (2019) 669–681
https://doi.org/10.1016/j.psc.2019.08.005
0193-953X/19/Published by Elsevier Inc.

the computer screen instead of looking at their patients and have resulted in physicians needing to spend hours after work catching up on charting.[3] As a result, physicians consistently rank EMRs as one of their top complaints.[1,4]

Physicians unfortunately had little say in the implementation of the EMR. When the HITECH Act introduced meaningful use incentives to increase EMR adoption on a national scale, many institutions required their physicians to start using EMRs without soliciting sufficient feedback from physicians. Furthermore, training for the product was minimal, often lasting only a few hours to a few days. When EMR upgrades are rolled out, often quarterly, physicians can be caught off-guard by unexpected changes in the user interface, disrupting workflows that they had created to adapt to previous upgrades and design changes.

This history has caused a strained and complicated relationship between physicians and the EMR. In 2016, Medscape surveyed 15,285 physicians across more than 25 specialties, and 57% of respondents reported EMRs reduced face-to-face time with patients, and approximately half reported seeing less patients because of slower workflows.[3] At the same time, more than half reported that EMRs improved documentation (56%) and made it easier to locate patient information (57%).[3]

TECHNOLOGIES ARE ONLY AS GOOD AS THE ORGANIZATION'S IMPLEMENTATION

Historically, organizations viewed technology implementation as a business decision, not a clinical one. This has led to physicians often being excluded from the design, evaluation, and implementation of new technologies. Many studies indicate that technologies, such as EMRs and computerized physician order entry, have contributed to factors associated with physician burnout.[1,5,6,7,8] They increase clerical burden, create inefficiencies, decrease productivity, and erode the doctor-patient relationship.[1,2,9,10] However, many of these initial studies evaluated technologies that were not designed specifically for health care applications, making them ill-suited for integrating into physician workflows. In addition to physicians not being involved in the evaluation and decision to implement technologies, health care organizations also lack tools to appropriately assess the potential impact of technology on physician workflows, workloads, and well-being.

A NEED FOR A SYSTEMATIC FRAMEWORK TO EVALUATE THE IMPACT OF TECHNOLOGIES ON PHYSICIAN WELL-BEING

Research studies often lag far behind the pace at which new technologies become available, making it difficult for organizations to have access to reliable data and best practices on how to incorporate new technologies into their health systems. This problem is further exacerbated by the fact that there are few high-quality studies available on the impact of technology on physician health and well-being as described in several systematic reviews.[11-13] Therefore, health care organizations often lack the clinical data needed to make evidence-based decisions on how to implement new technologies, particularly in digital health.

THE UNIVERSITY OF CALIFORNIA TECHNOLOGY WELLNESS INDEX

The University of California Technology Wellness Index (UCTWI), which we have developed, offers a framework for efficiently evaluating the impact of a given technology on a clinician's well-being. Modeled on Stanford Medicine's WellMD Professional Fulfillment Index and the Institute for Healthcare Improvement's Quadruple Aim,[14-17] the UCTWI was developed as a tool to focus on evaluating technology's impact on physician well-being, because no other tool currently exists for this purpose. The tool is used to evaluate digital health technologies or changed workflows and clinical processes.

Because the speed of innovation often outpaces the ability to evaluate each technology in a timely, academically rigorous way, the UCTWI provides organizations with an efficient, systematic, physician-centered framework for assessing the potential impact of new technologies on physician burnout and well-being. The UCTWI aims to evaluate technologies and their impact on physician well-being across three major categories: (1) productivity, (2) lifestyle, and (3) meaning (**Fig. 1**). Each category has subcategories that are assessed individually (**Table 1**). By optimizing these variables, organizations can introduce technologies and related processes to maximize the well-being of their physicians and the care of their patients.

Productivity

Physicians value being productive, and for many physicians, being efficient in their work translates to treating more patients. Technologies can aid in helping physicians see more patients during the day through two major mechanisms: improving their efficiency and/or reducing nonclinical work (ie, increasing time for clinical work). **Table 2** provides some examples of how various interventions have affected physician

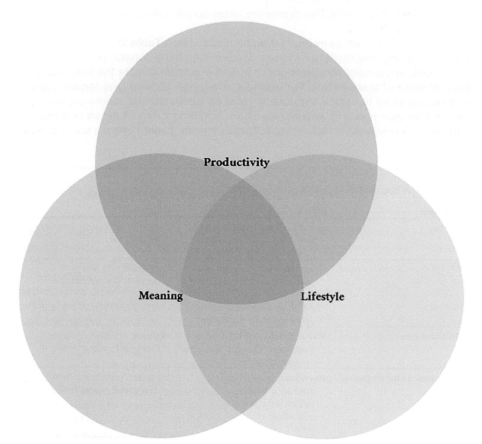

Fig. 1. University of California Technology wellness index: primary categories.

Table 1
University of California Technology Wellness Index: scoring rubric

Category	Subcategory	Score
Productivity	*Efficiency*: Does the technology affect the physician's overall efficiency in clinical and nonclinical work?	0/1
	Clinical Productivity: Does the technology allow the physician to spend less time on nonclinical work?	0/1
Meaning	*Patient Engagement*: Does this increase/decrease the proportion of time and the ease that the physician spends engaging with patients?	0/1
	Case Mix: Does the technology enable the physician to have more control over the case mix across their patient panel?	0/1
	Teamwork: Does the technology create a more collaborative work environment?	0/1
Lifestyle	*Time*: Does the technology free up physician time away from work?	0/1
	Independence: Does the technology increase independence, schedule flexibility, and autonomy for the physician?	0/1
	Financial: Does this affect the physician's income?	0/1
UCTWI Score		0–8

efficiency and productivity. This domain includes nonclinical activities, such as teaching and research.

Some activities, such as multifactor authentication (see **Table 2**), are necessary for security reasons, and these nonwellness factors need to be considered when making responsible implementation decisions. It is also important to note the temporal variance of some of these effects. For example, many new technologies require training and getting used to, which temporarily reduces efficiency and harms productivity. The organization needs to evaluate the short- and long-term outcomes of efficiency and net productivity when making impact assessments. **Table 1** offers a scoring rubric

Table 2
Positive and negative examples of efficiency of practice

Example	Effect	Outcome
Scribes	Scribes reduce the amount of time physicians need to spend charting in the EHR.	Increased efficiency, increased productivity
Multifactor authentication	Physicians have to type in a password and enter a long code that is texted to their cellphone increasing time it takes to log in to the EHR.	Decreased efficiency, decreased productivity
Telemedicine	Physicians do not have to walk from room to room reducing nonclinical time.	Reduced nonclinical work, increased productivity
Insurance authorizations	Physicians need to call insurance to get authorization for a procedure reducing clinical time.	Increased nonclinical work, decreased productivity

Abbreviation: EHR, electronic health record.

that is used for short- and long-term timeframes to evaluate the potential impact of introducing a new technology on physician productivity.

Meaning

Physicians gain intrinsic satisfaction and fulfillment from treating patients and building meaningful relationships with them.[17] Many physicians value the opportunity to get to know the patient, build rapport, and learn about their lives beyond the immediate clinical context, often resulting in improved patient engagement and outcomes.[18] Although clinical interactions have become more checklist-oriented because of time constraints and increased patient quotas, fortunately, technologies can help to improve patient engagement by increasing the amount of time physicians can spend interacting with their patients.

Many physicians also value having variety in their patient panels, whereas other physicians may prefer seeing specific patient populations that are rare and difficult to find. Case mix can have a strong impact on the physician finding meaning and fulfillment in their practice, and this needs to be assessed carefully and on a case-by-case basis. Technologies, such as telemedicine, eliminate geographic proximity as a barrier to seeing the patient, opening new possibilities for optimizing case mix tailored to each physician's preference.

Lifestyle

Physicians are increasingly valuing work-life balance as much as their income. An increasing proportion of physicians are working for large health systems as salaried employees, and working for small- to medium-sized practices is decreasing.[19–21] This has contributed to physicians having less independence in their practice, working in more regimented organizations that limit the physician's autonomy and flexibility.

Technologies, such as telepsychiatry and tele-ICU, have allowed physicians and nursing staff to have more flexibility in their work arrangements.[22] Technologies can also help increase income for physicians by increasing their productivity, offering more flexibility in living location/expenses, and increasing the catchment area of their services. They can also help to free up more time to dedicate to personal activities, such as travel, family, and hobbies. Therefore, technologies should be assessed in terms of impact on income, independence, and personal time as key factors in promoting a healthy lifestyle (see **Table 1**).

CASES

We present example cases demonstrating how UCTWI is used to score and evaluate the potential impact of new technologies on physician well-being. The process of using UCTWI and analyzing each subdomain could be as illuminating as the score itself. Because many of these issues are easily overlooked by an organization, one of the biggest values of using UCTWI may be the consistent, systematic assessment of each subdomain to ensure that a physician-centered perspective has been considered.

Transitioning to a New Electronic Medical Records System

In this example, a small psychiatric practice is evaluating whether to transition to a new EMR system with features that would aid in maximizing billing codes for each encounter. Because technologies often require time for physicians to familiarize themselves with the new product, often, there is a loss of productivity in the beginning. However, some technologies can yield net efficiencies and increased productivity over the long-term, improving physician well-being. This case highlights the utility of UCTWI across different timeframes of technology implementation. **Table 3** shows a UCTWI score of 0 in the short-term, likely resulting in a negative effect on physician well-being. However, this effect is temporary, and as the physicians get more familiar with the new EMR system, they realize that it is much easier to use than the previous one, decreasing charting time, and increasing practice revenue by using the new features that help with maximizing billing for each patient. **Table 3** shows a UCTWI score of 4 in the long-term indicating a positive effect on physician well-being. This example demonstrates the temporal effects of technology on physician health and also highlights how UCTWI is used as a relative scale to compare the effects of technology across different timeframes.

Synchronous Telepsychiatry

Telepsychiatry is now an established form of mental health care.[22] Many studies have demonstrated that it meets all appropriate standards of psychiatric care, and some studies have shown that telepsychiatry may be more effective than in-person consultations for certain groups of patients, such as children, adults with post-traumatic stress disorder or anxiety disorders, and correctional inmates.[23–25] Many patients now choose to receive their care in this hybrid manner that can be significantly better for them and for their providers than being seen exclusively in the clinic office for numerous reasons.[26]

Telepsychiatry is a well-studied technology, and in these cases, it is strongly recommended that data from the literature are incorporated into determining the UCTWI scores for each subcategory. Firstly, telemedicine consultations save time for the provider. It is easier to type notes at the same time as talking to the patient using telemedicine because it is socially much more appropriate to do this while maintaining eye contact via video. This can save several minutes of provider time per consultation, allowing more time to be spent with patients, and/or less time completing notes after

Table 3		
UCWTI for new EMR system (short-term and long-term scores)		
Category	**Subcategory**	**Score**
Productivity	*Efficiency*: Does the technology affect the physician's overall efficiency in clinical and nonclinical work?	0 (short-term) 1 (long-term)
	Clinical Productivity: Does the technology allow the physician to spend less time on nonclinical work?	0 (short-term) 1 (long-term)
Meaning	*Patient Engagement*: Does this increase/decrease the proportion of time and the ease that the physician spends engaging with patients?	0 (short-term) 0 (long-term)
	Case Mix: Does the technology enable the physician to have more control over the case mix across their patient panel?	0 (short-term) 0 (long-term)
	Teamwork: Does the technology create a more collaborative work environment?	0 (short-term) 0 (long-term)
Lifestyle	*Time*: Does the technology free up physician time away from work?	0 (short-term) 1 (long-term)
	Independence: Does the technology increase independence, schedule flexibility, and autonomy for the physician?	0 (short-term) 0 (long-term)
	Financial: Does this affect the physician's income?	0 (short-term) 1 (long-term)
UCTWI Score		0 (short-term) 4 (long-term)

hours for the physician.[22] More time is also saved because patients do not need to come into a physical room and leave, which can also save several minutes from each consultation. Our estimates of savings between 5 and 7 minutes per consultation makes a massive difference to provider efficiency and reduces their stress markedly over the course of a single day.

Flexibility of time and workplace is also really important for providers' work-life balance and their well-being. Telemedicine saves travel time for physicians by allowing them to remotely assess the patient rather than traveling to the hospital. One study found that using telepsychiatry in pediatric emergency rooms reduced the need for psychiatry fellows to travel to the pediatric emergency room by 75%, saving them 2.22 hours per weekend call day.[27] Psychiatrists, especially young women with families, are frequently choosing to work from home, and also offering consultations to patients in the evenings or weekends, making life more convenient for them and their patients. By reducing or eliminating travel time and creating more flexibility in their schedules, telemedicine allows physicians to spend more time at home, resulting in a better work-life balance.

Improved clinical quality through teamwork and gaining additional information on patients is another big advantage of telepsychiatry.[28–30] Many psychiatrists are able to work more easily with primary care physicians, who may join the consultations on video, and with patients' families, especially when the patients are seen at home. Finally some psychiatrists use telepsychiatry to develop panels of patients who are in alignment with their specialty interest, perhaps working in several different health systems to see patients with specific disorders in which they are experts. Other providers like the extra safety that comes with video consultations, especially if dealing with potentially dangerous patients, such as in correctional systems.

Overall, we calculated a UCTWI score of 5 (**Table 4**), indicating that implementing telepsychiatry could have a positive effect on physician well-being.

Asynchronous Telepsychiatry

Asynchronous telepsychiatry (ATP) offers additional advantages for the provider that can positively impact physician well-being. With asynchronous consultations,

Table 4 UCWTI for synchronous telepsychiatry		
Category	**Subcategory**	**Score**
Productivity	*Efficiency:* Does the technology affect the physician's overall efficiency in clinical and nonclinical work?	1
	Clinical Productivity: Does the technology allow the physician to spend less time on nonclinical work?	0
Meaning	*Patient Engagement:* Does this increase/decrease the proportion of time and the ease that the physician spends engaging with patients?	1
	Case Mix: Does the technology enable the physician to have more control over the case mix across their patient panel?	1
	Teamwork: Does the technology create a more collaborative work environment?	1
Lifestyle	*Time:* Does the technology free up physician time away from work?	0
	Independence: Does the technology increase independence, schedule flexibility, and autonomy for the physician?	1
	Financial: Does this affect the physician's income?	0
UCTWI Score		5

psychiatrists can assess their patients with much more efficiency and flexibility because the patient's responses to interview questions are recorded and are reviewed by the psychiatrist at their convenience.[31,32] Therefore, ATP enables providers to integrate patient care into their work day with optimal flexibility and control, positively impacting multiple aspects of physician well-being including productivity and lifestyle. Compared with synchronous telepsychiatry, one disadvantage is that patients are not able to see their psychiatrist in real time, likely reducing patient engagement, although synchronous follow-up visits can be arranged if necessary. Some patients may prefer the ease, flexibility, and convenience of ATP because they do not have to wait for the physician to start their clinical encounter. Overall, we calculated a UCTWI score of 7 (**Table 5**), demonstrating a relative improvement in physician well-being compared with synchronous telepsychiatry (see **Table 4**).

Using Google Glass and a Virtual Scribe App

Scribes have been used to reduce the burden of charting on physicians. Technologies, such as Google Glass and Amazon's Alexa-powered Echo devices, have been used in the clinical setting to aid in transcribing and charting patient encounters. For example, Google Glass allows physicians to wear an eyeglass-like device on their head that is equipped with a microphone and video camera. Google Glass can transmit the audio of the patient encounter in real-time to a software that automatically transcribes the encounter into a medical chart. Such companies as Augmedix, Nuance's Virtual Scribing Services, and DeepScribe already offer these types of services. Furthermore, such devices as Google Glass can be distracting to the patient, which could negatively impact patient engagement, but we ultimately gave a score of 1 on Patient Engagement for this example. Overall, we calculated a UCTWI score of 3 (**Table 6**).

Using Virtual Reality to See Psychiatry Patients

Virtual reality (VR) could offer similar benefits to those discussed in the telepsychiatry section.[26,33–35] This is a good example where the implementation details significantly influence the UCTWI score and impact on physician well-being. As shown in studies

Table 5
UCTWI for asynchronous telepsychiatry

Category	Subcategory	Score
Productivity	*Efficiency*: Does the technology affect the physician's overall efficiency in clinical and nonclinical work?	1
	Clinical Productivity: Does the technology allow the physician to spend less time on nonclinical work?	1
Meaning	*Patient Engagement*: Does this increase/decrease the proportion of time and the ease that the physician spends engaging with patients?	0
	Case Mix: Does the technology enable the physician to have more control over the case mix across their patient panel?	1
	Teamwork: Does the technology create a more collaborative work environment?	1
Lifestyle	*Time*: Does the technology free up physician time away from work?	1
	Independence: Does the technology increase independence, schedule flexibility, and autonomy for the physician?	1
	Financial: Does this affect the physician's income?	1
UCTWI Score		7

Table 6
UCTWI for Google glass with virtual scribe technology

Category	Subcategory	Score
Productivity	*Efficiency*: Does the technology affect the physician's overall efficiency in clinical and nonclinical work?	1
	Clinical Productivity: Does the technology allow the physician to spend less time on nonclinical work?	1
Meaning	*Patient Engagement*: Does this increase/decrease the proportion of time and the ease that the physician spends engaging with patients?	1
	Case Mix: Does the technology enable the physician to have more control over the case mix across their patient panel?	0
	Teamwork: Does the technology create a more collaborative work environment?	0
Lifestyle	*Time*: Does the technology free up physician time away from work?	0
	Independence: Does the technology increase independence, schedule flexibility, and autonomy for the physician?	0
	Financial: Does this affect the physician's income?	0
UCTWI Score		3

on telepsychiatry, VR could be a more intimate setting with the added protection offered by using avatars instead of real faces, particularly for adults with anxiety or post-traumatic stress disorder.[36] VR could provide physicians with increased control and flexibility over their schedule and case mix because they could be seeing patients from any location. It could offer even more flexibility than telemedicine because it would not require a professional backdrop or setting without video. Virtual or human scribes could also be incorporated into VR visits, which could improve physician efficiency and productivity, but we gave both scores of 0 in this example, assuming the physician would still chart on their own. Overall, we calculated a UCTWI score of 5, but depending on the design and implementation, a score of 8 could be achieved by increasing efficiency, productivity, and income for the psychiatrist (**Table 7**).

Table 7
UCTWI for psychiatry VR

Category	Subcategory	Score
Productivity	*Efficiency*: Does the technology affect the physician's overall efficiency in clinical and nonclinical work?	0
	Clinical Productivity: Does the technology allow the physician to spend less time on nonclinical work?	0
Meaning	*Patient Engagement*: Does this increase/decrease the proportion of time and the ease that the physician spends engaging with patients?	1
	Case Mix: Does the technology enable the physician to have more control over the case mix across their patient panel?	1
	Teamwork: Does the technology create a more collaborative work environment?	1
Lifestyle	*Time*: Does the technology free up physician time away from work?	1
	Independence: Does the technology increase independence, schedule flexibility, and autonomy for the physician?	1
	Financial: Does this affect the physician's income?	0
UCTWI Score		5

Table 8
UCTWI for remote monitoring app for bipolar patients

Category	Subcategory	Score
Productivity	*Efficiency*: Does the technology affect the physician's overall efficiency in clinical and nonclinical work?	1
	Clinical Productivity: Does the technology allow the physician to spend less time on nonclinical work?	0
Meaning	*Patient Engagement*: Does this increase/decrease the proportion of time and the ease that the physician spends engaging with patients?	1
	Case Mix: Does the technology enable the physician to have more control over the case mix across their patient panel?	0
	Teamwork: Does the technology create a more collaborative work environment?	1
Lifestyle	*Time*: Does the technology free up physician time away from work?	0
	Independence: Does the technology increase independence, schedule flexibility, and autonomy for the physician?	0
	Financial: Does this affect the physician's income?	0
UCTWI Score		3

Introducing a Remote Monitoring App for Bipolar Patients

Mobile technologies, such as smartphone apps, can provide physicians with valuable clinical data beyond the clinical setting. Apps have been developed for remote mood and activity monitoring for patients who are bipolar and for numerous other psychiatric and nonpsychiatric conditions.[37–40] A remote monitoring app for patients who are bipolar could help improve efficiency of psychiatrists during the patient encounter because reliable data on mood and other symptoms could be readily available before and during the appointment. It could also increase patient engagement because psychiatrists could review and analyze the data together with the patient, and it could create a sense of teamwork and camaraderie with the patient and potentially other providers who could access the data to manage the patient more holistically. Overall, a UCTWI score of 3 indicates a positive effect on physician well-being (**Table 8**).

LIMITATIONS

We have developed UCTWI as a guide for health care organizations looking for a tool and framework for systematically assessing the impact of technology on physician burnout and well-being. We expect that this tool will warrant case-specific adjustments to accommodate different environments and use cases. Because burnout is multifactorial and context-dependent, organizations are best suited to use their own assumptions and modify UCTWI to fit their clinical context.[41–43]

UCTWI has not been tested across different settings, such as varying organization size, specialty, and type of technology. More studies are needed to assess its validity and reliability across a broad range of use cases. We anticipate that one of the immediate benefits from using UCTWI is the systematic process of analyzing factors related to physician burnout and well-being and the discussion that ensues from the process.

SUMMARY

Technologies have significant potential to promote physician well-being and reduce burnout if evaluated and implemented appropriately. Technologies can improve quality of care, reduce administrative burdens, enhance physician autonomy, and support practice flexibility while saving costs for the health care system.

Because innovation almost always outpaces research and policies, organizations must develop efficient methods to systematically evaluate the potential impact of new technologies and changed processes on the well-being of their physicians, and on patient outcomes. As the practice of medicine continues to evolve with new technologies, more data, and a new generation of Millennials becoming practitioners, organizational leaders will play a critical role in listening to their physicians, engaging with diverse groups of practitioners, and promoting a culture of wellness that is nimble and responsive.

Technology at its core is a capability, neither good nor bad. It is our responsibility to apply technology in a manner that enhances medical practice, improves patient care, and supports physician health and well-being. Despite the increasing adoption of technology into medical practice, the benefits that technology can offer to physician health remain largely untapped. It is time to start evaluating the impact of health technologies on physician well-being using tools, such as the UCTWI described here.

REFERENCES

1. Shanafelt TD, Dyrbye LN, Sinsky C, et al. Relationship between clerical burden and characteristics of the electronic environment with physician burnout and professional satisfaction. Mayo Clin Proc 2016;91(7):836–48.

2. Verghese A. How tech can turn doctors into clerical workers. The New York Times 2018. Available at: https://www.nytimes.com/interactive/2018/05/16/magazine/health-issue-what-we-lose-with-data-driven-medicine.html. Accessed July 23, 2018.

3. Peckham C, Kane L, Rosensteel S. Medscape EHR Report 2016. Medscape 2016. Available at: https://www.medscape.com/features/slideshow/public/ehr2016. Accessed March 2, 2019.

4. Collier R. Electronic health records contributing to physician burnout. CMAJ 2017;189(45):E1405–6.

5. Cresswell KM, Bates DW, Williams R, et al. Evaluation of medium-term consequences of implementing commercial computerized physician order entry and clinical decision support prescribing systems in two 'early adopter' hospitals. J Am Med Inform Assoc 2014;21(e2):e194–202.

6. Gray A, Fernandes CMB, Aarsen KV, et al. The impact of computerized provider order entry on emergency department flow. CJEM 2016;18(4):264–9.

7. Schiff GD, Amato MG, Eguale T, et al. Computerised physician order entry-related medication errors: analysis of reported errors and vulnerability testing of current systems. BMJ Qual Saf 2015;24(4):264–71.

8. Bastani A, Walch R, Todd B, et al. 253: computerized prescriber order entry decreases patient satisfaction and emergency physician productivity. Ann Emerg Med 2010;56(3):S83–4.

9. West CP, Dyrbye LN, Shanafelt TD. Physician burnout: contributors, consequences and solutions. J Intern Med 2018;283(6):516–29.

10. Ehrenfeld JM, Wanderer JP. Technology as friend or foe? Do electronic health records increase burnout? Curr Opin Anaesthesiol 2018;31(3):357–60.

11. Mackintosh N, Terblanche M, Maharaj R, et al. Telemedicine with clinical decision support for critical care: a systematic review. Syst Rev 2016;5:176.

12. Venkataraman R, Ramakrishnan N. Outcomes related to telemedicine in the intensive care unit: what we know and would like to know. Crit Care Clin 2015;31(2): 225–37.

13. Ramnath VR, Ho L, Maggio LA, et al. Centralized monitoring and virtual consultant models of Tele-ICU care: a systematic review. Telemed J E Health 2014; 20(10):936–61.

14. WellMD Center. WellMD. Available at: https://wellmd.stanford.edu/center1.html. Accessed March 7, 2019.

15. Bodenheimer T, Sinsky C. From triple to quadruple aim: care of the patient requires care of the provider. Ann Fam Med 2014;12(6):573–6.

16. Feeley D. The triple aim or the quadruple aim? Four points to help set your strategy. IHI Improv Blog; 2017. Available at: http://www.ihi.org/communities/blogs/the-triple-aim-or-the-quadruple-aim-four-points-to-help-set-your-strategy. Accessed August 22, 2018.

17. Trockel M, Bohman B, Lesure E, et al. A brief instrument to assess both burnout and professional fulfillment in physicians: reliability and validity, including correlation with self-reported medical errors, in a sample of resident and practicing physicians. Acad Psychiatry 2018;42(1):11–24.

18. Parish MB, Fazio S, Chan S, et al. Managing psychiatrist-patient relationships in the digital age: a summary review of the impact of technology-enabled care on clinical processes and rapport. Curr Psychiatry Rep 2017;19(11):90.

19. Nakagawa K, Kvedar J, Yellowlees P. Retail outlets using telehealth pose significant policy questions for health care. Health Aff (Millwood) 2018;37(12):2069–75.

20. Welch WP, Cuellar AE, Stearns SC, et al. Proportion of physicians in large group practices continued to grow in 2009–11. Health Aff (Millwood) 2013;32(9): 1659–66.

21. Peterson LE, Baxley E, Jaén CR, et al. Fewer family physicians are in solo practices. J Am Board Fam Med 2015;28(1):11–2.

22. American Psychiatric Association. In: Yellowlees P, Shore JH, editors. Telepsychiatry and health technologies: a guide for mental health professionals. 1st edition. Arlington (VA): American Psychiatric Association Publishing; 2018.

23. Hilty DM, Rabinowitz T, McCarron RM, et al. An update on telepsychiatry and how it can leverage collaborative, stepped, and integrated services to primary care. Psychosomatics 2018;59(3):227–50.

24. Hilty DM, Ferrer DC, Parish MB, et al. The effectiveness of telemental health: a 2013 review. Telemed J E Health 2013;19(6):444–54.

25. Hilty DM, Yellowlees PM, Cobb HC, et al. Models of telepsychiatric consultation–liaison service to rural primary care. Psychosomatics 2006;47(2):152–7.

26. Yellowlees P, Richard Chan S, Burke Parish M. The hybrid doctor-patient relationship in the age of technology: Telepsychiatry consultations and the use of virtual space. Int Rev Psychiatry 2015;27(6):476–89.

27. Reliford A, Adebanjo B. Use of telepsychiatry in pediatric emergency room to decrease length of stay for psychiatric patients, improve resident on-call burden, and reduce factors related to physician burnout. Telemed J E Health 2018. https://doi.org/10.1089/tmj.2018.0124.

28. Chu-Weininger MYL, Wueste L, Lucke JF, et al. The impact of a tele-ICU on provider attitudes about teamwork and safety climate. Qual Saf Health Care 2010;19(6).

29. Hoonakker PLT, Pecanac KE, Brown RL, et al. Virtual collaboration, satisfaction and trust between nurses in the tele-ICU and ICUs: results of a multi-level analysis. J Crit Care 2017;37:224–9.

30. Bettinelli M, Lei Y, Beane M, et al. Does robotic telerounding enhance nurse–physician collaboration satisfaction about care decisions? Telemed J E Health 2015;21(8):637–43.
31. Yellowlees P, Burke Parish M, González Á, et al. Asynchronous telepsychiatry: a component of stepped integrated care. Telemed J E Health 2018;24(5):375–8.
32. Chan S, Li L, Torous J, et al. Review of use of asynchronous technologies incorporated in mental health care. Curr Psychiatry Rep 2018;20(10):85.
33. Maghazil A, Yellowlees P. Novel approaches to clinical care in mental health: from asynchronous telepsychiatry to virtual reality. In: Lech M, Song I, Yellowlees P, et al, editors. Mental health informatics. Studies in computational intelligence. Berlin: Springer Berlin Heidelberg; 2014. p. 57–78.
34. Hilty DM, Alverson DC, Alpert JE, et al. Virtual reality, telemedicine, web and data processing innovations in medical and psychiatric education and clinical care. Acad Psychiatry 2006;30(6):528–33.
35. Riva G, Gamberini L. Virtual reality in telemedicine. Telemed J E Health 2000;6(3): 327–40.
36. Parsons TD, Rizzo AA. Affective outcomes of virtual reality exposure therapy for anxiety and specific phobias: a meta-analysis. J Behav Ther Exp Psychiatry 2008;39(3):250–61.
37. Saunders KEA, Bilderbeck AC, Panchal P, et al. Experiences of remote mood and activity monitoring in bipolar disorder: a qualitative study. Eur Psychiatry 2017;41: 115–21.
38. Osmani V, Maxhuni A, Grünerbl A, et al. Monitoring Activity of Patients with Bipolar Disorder Using Smart Phones. The 11th International Conference on Advances in Mobile Computing & Multimedia. MoMM '13. New York, NY 2013;85. 85–85:92.
39. Martínez-Pérez B, de la Torre-Díez I, López-Coronado M, et al. Mobile apps in cardiology: review. JMIR MHealth UHealth 2013;1(2). https://doi.org/10.2196/mhealth.2737.
40. Semple JL, Sharpe S, Murnaghan ML, et al. Using a mobile app for monitoring post-operative quality of recovery of patients at home: a feasibility study. JMIR MHealth UHealth 2015;3(1). https://doi.org/10.2196/mhealth.3929.
41. Abedini NC, Stack SW, Goodman JL, et al. "It's Not Just Time Off": A Framework for Understanding Factors Promoting Recovery From Burnout Among Internal Medicine Residents. J Grad Med Educ 2017;10(1):26–32.
42. Shanafelt TD, Noseworthy JH. Executive Leadership and Physician Well-being: Nine Organizational Strategies to Promote Engagement and Reduce Burnout. Mayo Clin Proc. 2017;92(1):129–46.
43. Erickson SM, Rockwern B, Koltov M, et al. Medical Practice and Quality Committee of the American College of Physicians. Putting Patients First by Reducing Administrative Tasks in Health Care: A Position Paper of the American College of Physicians. Ann Intern Med 2017;166(9):659–61.

UNITED STATES POSTAL SERVICE®

Statement of Ownership, Management, and Circulation (All Periodicals Publications Except Requester Publications)

1. Publication Title	2. Publication Number	3. Filing Date
PSYCHIATRIC CLINICS OF NORTH AMERICA	000 – 703	9/18/2019

4. Issue Frequency	5. Number of Issues Published Annually	6. Annual Subscription Price
MAR, JUN, SEP, DEC	4	$332.00

7. Complete Mailing Address of Known Office of Publication (Not printer) (Street, city, county, state, and ZIP+4®)

ELSEVIER INC.
230 Park Avenue, Suite 800
New York, NY 10169

Contact Person
STEPHEN R. BUSHING

Telephone (Include area code)
215-239-3688

8. Complete Mailing Address of Headquarters or General Business Office of Publisher (Not printer)

ELSEVIER INC.
230 Park Avenue, Suite 800
New York, NY 10169

9. Full Names and Complete Mailing Addresses of Publisher, Editor, and Managing Editor (Do not leave blank)

Publisher (Name and complete mailing address)

TAYLOR BALL, ELSEVIER INC.
1600 JOHN F KENNEDY BLVD. SUITE 1800
PHILADELPHIA, PA 19103-2899

Editor (Name and complete mailing address)

LAUREN BOYLE, ELSEVIER INC.
1600 JOHN F KENNEDY BLVD. SUITE 1800
PHILADELPHIA, PA 19103-2899

Managing Editor (Name and complete mailing address)

PATRICK MANLEY, ELSEVIER INC.
1600 JOHN F KENNEDY BLVD. SUITE 1800
PHILADELPHIA, PA 19103-2899

10. Owner (Do not leave blank. If the publication is owned by a corporation, give the name and address of the corporation immediately followed by the names and addresses of all stockholders owning or holding 1 percent or more of the total amount of stock. If not owned by a corporation, give the names and addresses of the individual owners. If owned by a partnership or other unincorporated firm, give its name and address as well as those of each individual owner. If the publication is published by a nonprofit organization, give its name and address.)

Full Name	Complete Mailing Address
WHOLLY OWNED SUBSIDIARY OF REED/ELSEVIER, US HOLDINGS	1600 JOHN F KENNEDY BLVD. SUITE 1800 PHILADELPHIA, PA 19103-2899

11. Known Bondholders, Mortgagees, and Other Security Holders Owning or Holding 1 Percent or More of Total Amount of Bonds, Mortgages, or Other Securities. If none, check box ▶ ☐ None

Full Name	Complete Mailing Address
N/A	

12. Tax Status (For completion by nonprofit organizations authorized to mail at nonprofit rates) (Check one)
The purpose, function, and nonprofit status of this organization and the exempt status for federal income tax purposes:
☒ Has Not Changed During Preceding 12 Months
☐ Has Changed During Preceding 12 Months (Publisher must submit explanation of change with this statement)

PS Form 3526, July 2014 [Page 1 of 4 (see instructions page 4)] PSN: 7530-01-000-9931   PRIVACY NOTICE: See our privacy policy on www.usps.com.

---

13. Publication Title			14. Issue Date for Circulation Data Below	
PSYCHIATRIC CLINICS OF NORTH AMERICA			JUNE 2019	

15. Extent and Nature of Circulation			Average No. Copies Each Issue During Preceding 12 Months	No. Copies of Single Issue Published Nearest to Filing Date
a. Total Number of Copies (Net press run)			211	207
b. Paid Circulation (By Mail and Outside the Mail)	(1)	Mailed Outside-County Paid Subscriptions Stated on PS Form 3541 (include paid distribution above nominal rate, advertiser's proof copies, and exchange copies)	92	99
	(2)	Mailed In-County Paid Subscriptions Stated on PS Form 3541 (include paid distribution above nominal rate, advertiser's proof copies, and exchange copies)	0	0
	(3)	Paid Distribution Outside the Mails Including Sales Through Dealers and Carriers, Street Vendors, Counter Sales, and Other Paid Distribution Outside USPS®	58	71
	(4)	Paid Distribution by Other Classes of Mail Through the USPS (e.g., First-Class Mail®)	0	0
c. Total Paid Distribution (Sum of 15b (1), (2), (3), and (4))			150	170
d. Free or Nominal Rate Distribution (By Mail and Outside the Mail)	(1)	Free or Nominal Rate Outside-County Copies included on PS Form 3541	48	21
	(2)	Free or Nominal Rate In-County Copies Included on PS Form 3541	0	0
	(3)	Free or Nominal Rate Copies Mailed at Other Classes Through the USPS (e.g., First-Class Mail)	0	0
	(4)	Free or Nominal Rate Distribution Outside the Mail (Carriers or other means)	0	0
e. Total Free or Nominal Rate Distribution (Sum of 15d (1), (2), (3) and (4))			48	21
f. Total Distribution (Sum of 15c and 15e)			198	191
g. Copies not Distributed (See Instructions to Publishers #4 (page 3))			13	16
h. Total (Sum of 15f and g)			211	207
i. Percent Paid (15c divided by 15f times 100)			75.76%	89.01%

* If you are claiming electronic copies, go to line 16 on page 3. If you are not claiming electronic copies, skip to line 17 on page 3.

16. Electronic Copy Circulation		Average No. Copies Each Issue During Preceding 12 Months	No. Copies of Single Issue Published Nearest to Filing Date
a. Paid Electronic Copies	▶		
b. Total Paid Print Copies (Line 15c) + Paid Electronic Copies (Line 16a)	▶		
c. Total Print Distribution (Line 15f) + Paid Electronic Copies (Line 16a)	▶		
d. Percent Paid (Both Print & Electronic Copies) (16b divided by 16c × 100)	▶		

☒ I certify that 50% of all my distributed copies (electronic and print) are paid above a nominal price.

17. Publication of Statement of Ownership

☒ If the publication is a general publication, publication of this statement is required. Will be printed in the DECEMBER 2019 issue of this publication.   ☐ Publication not required.

18. Signature and Title of Editor, Publisher, Business Manager, or Owner	Date
STEPHEN R. BUSHING - INVENTORY DISTRIBUTION CONTROL MANAGER	9/18/2019

I certify that all information furnished on this form is true and complete. I understand that anyone who furnishes false or misleading information on this form or who omits material or information requested on the form may be subject to criminal sanctions (including fines and imprisonment) and/or civil sanctions (including civil penalties).

PS Form 3526, July 2014 (Page 3 of 4)   PRIVACY NOTICE: See our privacy policy on www.usps.com.

Moving?

Make sure your subscription moves with you!

To notify us of your new address, find your **Clinics Account Number** (located on your mailing label above your name), and contact customer service at:

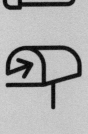

Email: **journalscustomerservice-usa@elsevier.com**

800-654-2452 (subscribers in the U.S. & Canada)
314-447-8871 (subscribers outside of the U.S. & Canada)

Fax number: **314-447-8029**

Elsevier Health Sciences Division
Subscription Customer Service
3251 Riverport Lane
Maryland Heights, MO 63043

*To ensure uninterrupted delivery of your subscription, please notify us at least 4 weeks in advance of move.